DIRECT RELEASE MYOFASCIAL TECHNIQUE

For Churchill Livingstone

Senior Commissioning Editor: Sarena Wolfaard
Project Development Manager: Dinah Thom
Project Manager: Jane Dingwall
Designer: Judith Wright

DIRECT RELEASE MYOFASCIAL TECHNIQUE

AN ILLUSTRATED GUIDE FOR PRACTITIONERS

Michael Stanborough BA MA

Certified Advanced Rolfer; Director, Stanborough Educational Group, Blackburn, Victoria, Australia; Full Instructor, Rolf Institute, Boulder, Colorado, USA

Forewords by

Robert Schleip MA

Faculty member of the Rolf Institute and of the European Rolfing Association, Munich, Germany

Peter J. O'Reilly MD

Certified Rolfer; Board Certified, American Board of Anesthesiology, Bozeman, Montana, USA

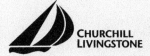
CHURCHILL
LIVINGSTONE

EDINBURGH LONDON NEW YORK OXFORD PHILADELPHIA ST LOUIS SYDNEY TORONTO 2004

CHURCHILL LIVINGSTONE
An imprint of Elsevier Limited

First published 2004

ISBN 0 443 07390 2

British Library Cataloguing in Publication Data
A catalogue record for this book is available from the British Library

Library of Congress Cataloging in Publication Data
A catalog record for this book is available from the Library of Congress

Notice
Medical knowledge is constantly changing. Standard safety precautions must be followed, but as new research and clinical experience broaden our knowledge, changes in treatment and drug therapy may become necessary or appropriate. Readers are advised to check the most current product information provided by the manufacturer of each drug to be administered to verify the recommended dose, the method and duration of administration, and contraindications. It is the responsibility of the practitioner, relying on experience and knowledge of the patient, to determine dosages and the best treatment for each individual patient. Neither the publishers nor the author will be liable for any loss or damage of any nature occasioned to or suffered by any person acting or refraining from acting as a result of reliance on the material contained in this publication.

The Publisher

Transferred to Digital Print 2009

The
Publisher's
policy is to use
**paper manufactured
from sustainable forests**

Printed and bound in Great Britain by
CPI Antony Rowe, Chippenham and Eastbourne

CONTENTS

FOREWORDS

There are books which offer just another spin on a common subject, maybe with a different emphasis than previous authors, yet which add nothing substantially new to the vast field of literature that is already available in the field of manual therapies. The book which you hold in your hands, dear reader, clearly belongs to a different kind. It is the first time that an internationally respected teacher of deep tissue work offers an easy to follow and clearly organized manual for direct myofascial techniques.

Among the field of myofascial release, two main streams can be described. There are the more recent schools of '*indirect release*', which have been influenced by Lawrence Jones, Rolin Becker, Jean Pierre Barral and others. Their hands tend to first 'go with' the direction of the somatic dysfunction, and then they allow the system to rewind itself from there. For example if the right shoulder of a client is chronically pulled forward, an indirect approach practitioner will manually support the shoulder going exactly in that forward direction until some release is felt towards a new and less contracted direction. Naturally these approaches tend to be experienced as more gentle and less intrusive by the client. Yet they also tend to have their limits (or need to be repeated for years) in many cases of severe tissue shortening or adhesion. Several excellent courses, textbooks and manuals are easily available on these techniques.

On the other side are the '*direct release*' techniques, in which the practitioner works directly towards the preferred and more healthy direction. To loosen a tight myofascial area, the practitioner's hands or elbow slowly sink directly into the tightened myofascial tissue. Often the client is then invited to contact the same place from the inside (via breathing or subtle joint movements) while the manual pressure is gradually increased (up to several pounds of pressure) until the tissue softens. For example in the client with the protracted shoulder, one might work directly on the tissues of pectoralis major or minor or on the ligaments around the coracoid process (see pp161–163) in order to release the shoulder directly out of its protracted pattern. This approach is often referred to as '*deep tissue work*' and tends to be seen among practitioners as more traditional. While being criticized as too violent and as 'old fashioned' by some, it is also experienced as magically powerful and as deeply profound by others. Most, yet not all, practitioners of this approach have been influenced by the work of Ida Rolf (1896–1979), founder of the Rolfing® method of structural integration, or by other schools of 'Structural Integration', 'Hellerwork', 'Postural Integration', etc., whose originators were inspired by Ida Rolf's work. Teaching of this approach has been more guarded, and up to now no authorized manual or 'how-to-do textbook' has been published.

Michael Stanborough chose to be the one 'who spills the beans' with this book. As you will quickly see, he spills the beans in a very thorough and professionally didactic manner. This is an historical step and is reminiscent of the change in the bodywork culture which John Upledger triggered with his first book on craniosacral therapy in 1983. Prior to that, the teaching of cranial osteopathy was mostly done behind closed doors in osteopathic colleges, and only after several years of more fundamental preparation. Upledger's book was therefore immensely criticized by many traditionally oriented osteopaths, as they had every reason to fear a dangerous increase of courses and treatments by not adequately trained practitioners. Of course this is also what has happened since then, and today it is not uncommon to find cranial osteopathic work being offered by lay people who learned this work in a weekend course. Yet on the other side of the coin, Upledger's book – and the resulting popularization of this approach – have led to a tremendous increase of international scientific research in this field as well as to new publications, conferences, discussions, concepts and unexpected insights.

I hope that Michael Stanborough is prepared for a similar upset against this book from many traditionally oriented representatives of his field. Their arguments are easy to anticipate and I believe that their warnings should not be taken lightly: this book may allow poorly trained and poorly motivated people to learn powerful deep tissue techniques in which their clients may be traumatized physically as well as psychologically. Yes, this danger will be there, due to the level of depth and the manual pressure which is sometimes involved in direct release deep tissue work. Nevertheless, if the beans are to be spilled – which I believe ought to happen anyway by one way or another in our rapidly changing culture – it makes a big difference how well this is done. And who does it.

Michael Stanborough is an authority in his field. He has been teaching this work for decades, plus he is a respected faculty member of the international Rolf Institute, which is considered by many of us a quality leader within this field. In reading through his manuscript, I have been reassured and impressed by how detailed the instructions and explanations are. On one side, the descriptions and accompanying pictures are so clear and easy to follow that it is possible to learn the basis of many of these techniques without any further personal instruction. Yet by working through this manual

the reader will also learn how evolved and refined this work can be. While this book will encourage the 'weekend warrior' practitioner types to look for professional training which teaches at the same thorough and intelligent level of instruction as is shown in this book, it will also be an invaluable asset for those more mature practitioners who already have a professional background in this work or in a related field within manual therapy.

What cannot be taught in written form is the important perceptual training. This includes the fascinating field of structural bodyreading, movement analysis, the refinement of palpatory touch for tissue responses, and the tracking of subtle responses of the autonomic nervous system in the client's body as well as in the practitioner's own body perception. Other aspects are the client–practitioner relationship and the strategic planning plus process oriented orchestration of a session or series of sessions. These are generally taught via personal instruction by experienced instructors. My prediction is that it will be exactly in these professional trainings that this book will soon become the most widely used textbook. As an instructor myself I have seen preliminary versions of some excerpts of this book being passed around among students as popular underground notes. And several students even approached me in a friendly manner about whether I could not supply them with regular handouts 'of this quality'. My reply was something like 'Do you have any idea how much work is behind each of these pages?!'. Well here it is, dear reader: a giant step forward in a modern and more user-friendly direction of learning and teaching this wonderful work.

Robert Schleip
Munich, Germany, 2004

This book is about direct technique myofascial release (MFR). It is a manual for anyone wanting to learn and incorporate this technique within a practice of manual therapy. Until now there has been a conspicuous absence of a textbook for direct technique MFR. What follows for the reader is a guide and workbook to which one can refer again and again. I have heard it said that it takes three to five years of experience before one gets really good at this technique. For anyone just beginning or

already started on that journey, this book will be a welcome companion. Almost as mysteriously as the eyes in the painting that seem to follow the observer, new material will seem to have been introduced into the text with each reading. Obviously it is the reader who has changed between readings. The Latin saying, *quidquid recipitur recipitur quo modo recipientis* (whatever is received is received according to the manner of the receiver), was never truer. In other words, a student is going to learn what they are ready to learn. It is this readiness which fluctuates.

This text offers the reader who has seen demonstrations of direct technique multiple chances to take in what they saw at progressively deeper levels. There are many times after a demonstration that I have wished that I could view it again. If learners are at the level where the information they need is how to contact the first layer of fascia ready to be worked, this author explains how to contact that specific layer. If the concern is with the relative position of the client and themselves, that information is easily accessed. For the students asking what their intention needs to be or even what they need to be thinking while they are working, this topic is covered. When students are ready to incorporate client movement into their work, they are guided in how to word the cues given to the client in a way that evokes movement with direction. The text has many layers of information available for all students of direct technique MFR wherever they are personally in their process of becoming really good practitioners.

For those interested in the finer nuances that can make a difference, this workbook is comprehensive and full of what I term 'pearls'. Pearls are suggestions, information, advice, tricks of the trade or shortcuts which make anything we do truly better and more effective. For the most part pearls are handed down by word of mouth from mentor to student, from master to novice, and from practitioner to practitioner. There are pearls between the covers of this book.

Not always proceeding in the manner or even direction we expect, learning does not always progress in a linear fashion, if you will, from point A to point B, from point B to point C, and so forth. Rather it seems we first grasp a few new details, then suddenly seem to have an insight making sense of the bigger picture, only to realize shortly thereafter that an old confusion has reintroduced itself, and the big picture is lost again. Not being able to see the forest for the trees can alternate with not being able to see the trees for the forest. Nowhere

is this more prevalent than when observing a demonstration of these techniques with a real client by a practitioner of 10, 15, 20 or more years of experience. The details of the work can be so overwhelming that the observer may later go blank when trying to duplicate what they have observed. What side of the client am I to stand on to work this part of the body? Which tool should I use? What am I thinking about? Or what should I be thinking about? What am I supposed to feel? In short, what am I doing? How do I stay connected with myself or with the client? All these questions can go through one's mind as one at the same time frantically attempts to take notes about the demonstration. I cannot tell you how many times I observed a demonstration of direct technique MFR, thought I completely understood what I needed to do, thinking I had a good sense of the big picture, only to be completely stymied by the details that I could not recall.

This text encompasses all the details so that with time, practice and experience one can become really good at direct technique myofascial release. Each presentation of the technique is simplified to its most basic elements of what pertains to the client, to the therapist, to the actual performance of the technique, and to methods of incorporating client movement. The commentaries are informative, thoughtful and practical. The division of chapters and subdivisions within chapters are completely user friendly for easy reference. Pediatric supplements are bonuses for anyone working with children. The author's approach is completely in agreement with the approach of the best of modern medical treatment of children. They are not just little adults for whom one simply downsizes adult techniques on a per kilogram basis. The techniques described are appropriate and specifically adapted for the child.

I pass on to the reader what Michael Stanborough passed on to me: enjoy.

Peter J. O'Reilly
Montana, USA, 2004

PREFACE

Until now there has been a conspicuous absence of a text that details the direct technique approach to myofascial release (MFR). Cranial, visceral and trigger point therapies all have elaborate texts that detail technique and rationale. This book is designed to provide a similar resource for those interested in exploring the breadth and depth of direct technique MFR.

In the past several years, various styles of MFR, originating from a number of sources, have become popular in the treatment of orthopedic and neurologic dysfunctions. MFR is also being used with that broad group in the population who fall into the category of having subclinical difficulties that nag and hinder, but do not disable. With this population there is a growing appreciation of the need to manage stress more effectively. This stress is often intuitively identified as an underlying cause of the failure to live at full function. It is very much my contention that direct technique MFR has a great deal to offer that population as well as those with true clinical difficulties. This is based on 20+ years of clinical observation.

Once the domain of alternative therapists, these various soft tissue techniques now enjoy popularity amongst manual therapists of all kinds – physical, occupational, massage and speech therapists, as well as many chiropractors and osteopaths; in short, anyone interested in providing comprehensive and useful hands-on therapy.

The principal approach that I employ in my classes and the most frequently described in this manual is the direct method of fascial release developed by Dr Ida Rolf. There are certainly other approaches that have significantly influenced my work but Dr Rolf's approach to directly engaging with fascial restriction and disorganization is at the core of this book. The question will arise; isn't this the Rolfing® method of Structural Integration? Or at least just plain old generic structural integration? The answer is a qualified no. Structural integration is a method informed by a philosophy regarding human posture and movement in the gravitational field. This book presents approaches to working with myofascia that a structural integration practitioner might use. But it does not attempt to teach the underlying philosophy of that method, nor the strategic protocols for achieving its goals. The material presented here is for all manual therapists.

The growing acceptance and use of direct technique MFR, along with other soft tissue approaches, is clearly a desirable development. The people who benefit from the dissemination of this knowledge are the clients who walk through our respective doors seeking help.

I am indebted to all of the pediatric therapists, and the children they work on, that I have taught over the years. Working with children has been heartwarming and fascinating. In many instances I have been fortunate to co-treat with very capable and creative therapists. Learning to integrate myofascial release into existing pediatric therapies enabled me to see more clearly the relationship between human structure and function. This insight has spilled over into all areas of my own practice.

This text was originally produced in response to students' continued requests for photos and descriptions of all the releases from the classes that I teach. While teaching, it was apparent that my hands had grown accustomed to doing things automatically. Being coaxed to recognize and record what I actually do as I work has had a number of rewards. One of them is this text. On the way to developing it, there have been numerous other benefits as well. I like to think my work is better for the close scrutiny my approaches have been given as I detailed them here. In bodywork, the notion that a picture is worth a thousand words is completely accurate. I sincerely hope this photographic manual will be useful and validate that idea.

Michael Stanborough
Victoria, Australia, 2004

ACKNOWLEDGEMENTS

Many people made this book possible. I would like firstly to express my deep appreciation to my teachers – Louis Schultz, Michael Shea, Stacey Mills, Annie Duggan, Jim Asher, Michael Salveson, Emmett Hutchins and Sally Klemm.

I am grateful to Robert Schleip who generously shares, through a variety of media, the knowledge he has gained as a result of decades of searching through material related to fascia, movement and human well-being. Thanks also to Beverly Veltman and Louise Horst who welcomed me into their pediatric clinics and shared their many insights into working with children. Of the many groups I have had the pleasure of presenting for, I am especially grateful to Dallas Easter Seal Society for Children for their support as I developed the pediatric application of this work. They demonstrate a cheerful consistency in promoting any work that may help the children in their care.

Thanks to friends: Fiona Wood for many things, especially the use of her sunny verandah, an excellent place to write, in Perth on several occasions; Barbralu Cohen of Words at Work in Boulder, Colorado, for her thoughts on making these particular words of mine work.

And my deep appreciation to that warrior of warriors, Chögyum Trungpa Rinpoche, for both leading from the front and pushing from behind, as needed.

Finally, my thanks to my family – to my children Liam and Farrah for love, humor and firm reminders that a computer is not the center of the universe. My deepest gratitude to Victoria – singer, teacher, visionary, mother and wife.

Michael Stanborough
Victoria, Australia, 2004

Section 1
THE BASICS

Chapter 1

INTRODUCTION

ABOUT ANATOMY WITHIN THIS BOOK

Defining which soft tissue structures belong to which region of the body is clearly not straightforward. Many muscles cross major joints and can potentially belong to two regions. In this workbook the reader will notice instances where structures have been included in one section when a case could just as easily be made for including them in another. Psoas is a trunk muscle but also a pelvic muscle and a leg muscle. Where should it be situated in this book? I've made it part of the pelvic work while an advanced approach to releasing it shows up in the trunk. The crest of the pelvis, on the other hand, shows up in the lower extremity because it relates so much to releasing all the tight structures of the lateral thigh. And so on. I've tried where possible to explain my thinking about these placements in the Comments section accompanying the description of each release. In truth, I don't think it's that big a deal. Our internal sense of body parts and their placement does not organize itself according to the textbooks. I don't think we should get too worried, other than to use it as a way to draw a convenient, pragmatic map.

The language of anatomy is one I can use to speak to the reader from a distance. When I say 'gluteus medius' we have a general agreement on the location of that muscle. If you do not know it, then every anatomy book in print will direct you to it. But if I say 'deep inner line' or 'superficial front line', you would have to read Tom Myers' excellent *Anatomy Trains*[1] to understand this reference. To talk about the jaw retinaculum you'd need to have read the equally useful *The Endless Web*.[2]

Both those books are worthwhile attempts to create a holistic anatomy. They each develop interesting schemas for understanding relationships in the body. This book is, in a sense, the 'applied' companion to both those texts. Still, we're left with the need to speak a language that we can have some agreement on, otherwise we've arrived at a postmodern language impasse without a way forward.

Buddhist descriptions of the nature of existence incorporate two views: relative and absolute. One might think that the absolute is better – 'I'll just study that view, thank you' – but in fact, we study one to more fully understand the other. For me, dissection reveals both discrete parts, incredible worlds unto themselves, as well as layers of connection. While this book orients itself by necessity to the parts, it is with the knowledge that there is also connection, continuity and wholeness.

TOUCH AND COMMUNICATION

Our thoughts, daydreams and images of our work, and ourselves at work, are major factors in determining the outcome of what we do as we work. As I see it, what we are occupied with at the level of imagination varies, depending on our professional label, the setting where we provide our services, our latest training and what our client's expectations are, to name just a very few influences. Family and culture of origin would be significant as well.

The possibilities of where and how we direct these dreams and formulations are numerous. However, a common thread can be found in all that we do in the touch therapies; namely, that we give expression to our intention through our hands.

Doing this work is enjoyable. I find it feels most like a well-honed extension of a deep ability to communicate through touch and very little like an attempt to stretch human rubber bands to a greater length. Once, when presenting myofascial release (MFR) to a group of doctors and chiropractors in Korea, we spent some time trying to define how I thought of this work. My complete lack of Korean and their good but somewhat limited English made this an interesting project. I was trying to point to my orientation as a somatics therapist, as opposed to a physical therapist, and not getting the point across too clearly. It was a good lesson in how different cultures view the importance of subjectivity. As a somatic therapist, I would say the subjective experience of the client is central to the therapy process. This orientation was clearly alien to them and we went around in a good-natured way as to why I thought the way I did. In the end I was delighted when one of the participants came to the enthusiastic conclusion that this MFR stuff is all about communication. Yes, yes, yes!

One aspect of somatic therapy is that the internal sensations and processes of the client are central to the process of therapy and education. Part of that process is to make visible the invisible. There is a sense of going on a voyage of discovery. Correction of musculoskeletal disorders will often but not always be an important part of the journey. In contrast, medical manual therapy might be defined as any corrections made to a client's body via the skillful interventions of a therapist. Measurements of change recorded by the therapist are central to this process. One approach is in the humanistic psychology domain while the other is part of the subject–object orientation of medicine.

In somatic therapy the practitioner deliberately explores his or her own inner experience during a treatment. They seek to model the state they are encouraging their client to explore. This is commonly known these days as embodiment. (If this type of exploration is appealing, then Chapter 4 will be of interest.) In medical manual therapy, the technique is applied to correct a problem and the state of the therapist is not considered pertinent to the interaction.

It is my hope that this book appeals to both groups. Personally, I observe that the distinctions are becoming less obvious. In Australia, for example, I notice many physiotherapists training as Feldenkrais practitioners while some massage therapists are heading to osteopathic school. Massage in the UK can now be studied at university level.

Times are a-changin'; boundaries are blurring and although some fundamentalists from each camp decry this development, to me it seems not only inevitable but also a sign of maturation. It's about finding a new edge that stimulates the creative mind.

Everyone who persists with myofascial release and develops a feedback loop that enables self-evaluation can become good at it. Feedback means the ability to gauge the effect of what is happening as you work. It is not external feedback via a client form, although one of those might be slightly helpful. It's about listening and paying attention to the relationship that is developing with an individual as we work with them.

As you put in the practice to get to the point where you are a good or even great practitioner, first and foremost do no harm to yourself by excess effort. It's amazingly common. I know many therapists (I've had my turn too) struggle with aches and pains brought on by their work. If you're aware of that threshold of effort and don't work past it, you can also be confident that you are not hurting your clients either. There's a whole section on the subject of how to work with maximum contact and minimal effort after this introduction. It's there because, as I mentioned, I've had my turn with occupational aches and pains.

INTEGRATION VERSUS DISINTEGRATION

In all professions the meaning of certain terms is taken for granted without a real appreciation of their actual definition. In manual therapies, the term 'integration' seems to have become just such a term. It shows up everywhere these days. What is actually being talked about when the term 'integration' is used? It sounds important – no-one wants to hang out a sign saying 'Disintegrative Therapy'. Moshe Feldenkrais called his body of work 'Functional Integration' and Dr Rolf named hers 'Structural Integration' (only later did her early students shift to calling it Rolfing®). Sharon Weislefish has developed 'Integrative Manual Therapy®' while Jack Painter uses the term 'Postural Integration' for his version of structural integration work. As a teacher and 20+ years practitioner of the Rolf® method of structural integration, I have used the term somewhat blindly myself.

A search on the Internet showed an impressive 121 000 listings when the words 'integration' and 'therapy' were typed into the Google search engine. Clearly linking the word to therapy is popular.

A trip to the dictionary is useful. (Don't panic, this is a short visit only.) *Webster's College Dictionary* defines integration as, amongst other things, '*1. An act or instance of incorporating or combining into a whole*' and, more usefully, even though it is from the domain of psychology, '*6. Psychol. The organization of the constituent elements of the personality into a coordinated, harmonious whole*'.

Both definitions give us insight into what we might aspire to with integration in body therapies. Even if we are not working within the kind of comprehensive framework of integration that Rolf and Feldenkrais developed, we might track the responses to direct technique myofascial release across a number of systems. Widening the scope of what we see as being affected by our manual therapy interventions will develop a fuller appreciation of integration and the potential for disintegration. People are complex beings, not simply biomechanical or biochemical entities that will one day be fully diagnosed and treated from within those two approaches alone. We are, at our disintegrated worst, a parcel of parts with numerous influences – biological, social, philosophical, biomechanical and so on – working to shape us into the people we are.

Back to the dictionary. '*The organization of the constituent elements of the personality into a coordinated, harmonious whole.*' Or we might say the organization of the constituent elements (be they psychic or corporeal) of a person into a harmonious whole.

It's not possible for any one somatic therapist to master every possible avenue of meaningful, therapeutic interaction with another person in one lifetime. Still, if we acknowledge that more systems than simply the myofascial are being affected as we work, as proposed in the following section, we can develop a sensitivity to and appreciation of a range of responses being made to what we are doing. At a simple level this might mean recognizing that the well-intended deep tissue work that made the client repeatedly wince and complain of pain was not the best therapy for them. It might actually activate the sympathetic nervous system (SNS), inflame tissue and create a feeling in the client that their experience of pain and possibly abuse at the hands of the

therapist was not listened to or considered important. Disassociation might become a strategy for tolerating future sessions. As the old communication theory saw goes, 'The response to what you say (do) is the meaning of it'.

Creating disintegration – disorganization of the person's constituent parts – is a real possibility in manual therapy. Yes, disintegration really does happen. Change isn't inherently desirable. To get that point across, one of my teachers once said, 'It's easy to change somebody. All you have to do is throw them down the stairs'. Mindless application of techniques without any appreciation of the person they are being applied to can lead to disintegration. Failure to be involved in a dynamic feedback loop as we're working, with the attendant lack of responsiveness, can do it. Even worse are the therapists who feel it is their role to counsel their clients on a range of important life issues while determining the basis for this unasked-for advice from poking and prodding into tight tissues. 'These neck muscles are tight – prod, poke – because you are not speaking out … you're not saying something you should say in your marriage. Perhaps you should get a divorce.' 'Have you been sexually abused? No? Your pelvis is awfully locked up … you've probably just repressed the memory … let's work on this … it's only painful because you are so tight.' Over the decades I've heard many tales about these kinds of hopefully well-intended but very questionable attempts to lend a psychological color to sessions.

This is not overtly a book about integrative ways of seeing and relating to the body. It's about a series of techniques, described as much as possible in terms that include a number of interactive elements, which can be utilized by a range of manual therapy practitioners in a broad variety of settings. Some will have a deliberate schema of integration in their background (Rolfing®, Hellerwork, Postural Integration, Feldenkrais, Sensory Integration, Neurodevelopmental Treatment and so on) while others who use this book will have a broad sense of integration in their work without naming that as its deliberate endeavor. Still others will be involved in rehabilitative settings where the workplace defines the scope of practice and the anatomy that can be worked on. Here there will perhaps be less scope for overt agendas of integration. Others will do largely corrective therapy via joint manipulation and mobilization, trigger point therapy and other procedures to influence local problems and pain. This book is intended for all these groups. It is my hope that the attitude to MFR described in this book will enable the work to be presented always in an orderly, organizing manner.

I tend to shift my foci on a seasonal basis, with the emphasis often determined by the latest training I've taken. I suspect we all tend to concentrate on new information and techniques until they are integrated and we make them our own. This sense of mastery generally involves practice, modification, rejection of some information and ongoing experimentation. The approach to working with soft tissue detailed in this book is not intended to imply a doctrinaire, 'this is the only way to do it' philosophy. I think there are other profoundly useful approaches to body therapy. It's just that until now no-one has truly organized direct technique myofascial release into a systematic workbook approach in the way visceral, cranial and other approaches have been.

PEDIATRIC APPLICATIONS

This book contains photos and illustrations of both adults and children being treated. The work on children is intended for pediatric therapists or experienced practitioners of other related therapies that have a pediatric application. I discourage parents with cerebral palsied children from attempting these releases on them. While these home help efforts are always well intended, this work requires a foundation of training in movement development, anatomy and physiology to be done safely. Furthermore, more is not better. It might seem a logical extension of the rationale behind the techniques to apply them very frequently for long-term disability. However, MFR for children with disabilities needs to be placed in a broad context of other therapies. It augments rather than replaces these approaches. A trained pediatric therapist will be able to determine how best to integrate these releases into existing protocols.

LAST THOUGHTS ...

All the talk of fascia, thixotropy, the autonomic nervous system and intrafascial mechanoreceptors that follows this introduction might cloud the fact that we work on people, not tissue. I hope not, as I believe any technical review should illuminate, and not blind, our view of the complex processes and concerns of the people we touch. Studying the relative view helps illuminate the big picture.

References

1. Myers T 2000 Anatomy trains. Churchill Livingstone, Edinburgh, UK
2. Schultz L, Feitis R 1996 The endless web. North Atlantic, Berkeley, CA

Chapter 2
DEVELOPING A HYPOTHETICAL MODEL

PRACTICE SEEKS THEORY

Myofascial release is a practice in search of a theory. Almost. By reviewing the histologic, mechanical, physiologic and neurologic aspects of connective tissue in general, and fascia in particular, a balance can be found between the enthusiastic clinical anecdotes that exist about the efficacy of myofascial release and a rational basis for understanding how the technique works.

Connective tissue is the most pervasive substance in the human body. For example, fascia, a specialized type of connective tissue, surrounds, invests and protects all the visceral and somatic structures of the body. The fascial sheaths entwined in and around muscle account for most of the immediate lengthening of muscle after stretching. Even with joint mobilization, the primary structures being affected are the joint capsules and the periarticular connective tissue – in other words, the soft connective tissues.

CONNECTIVE TISSUE

Connective tissue is generally divided into five principal groups:

- ordinary
- blood
- cartilage
- adipose
- bone.

Manual therapists are primarily interested in ordinary connective tissue which includes the subgroups of superficial and deep fascial sheaths, nerve and muscle sheaths, the supporting framework of internal organs, aponeuroses, ligaments, joint capsules, periosteum and tendons.

Cells

All connective tissues consist of cells and extracellular matrix (ECM). The cells, primarily fibroblasts, are responsible for producing the ECM. Macrophages and histiocytes are also found in connective tissue and are involved in phagocytosing waste and foreign matter. Also present are mast cells, responsible for producing histamine and heparin, and plasma cells, which are mostly found in pathologic situations. With the exception of fibroblasts, all these cells are involved in the reticuloendothelial system.

Imagine a body with all the cells removed. What would remain? An amorphous pile of ... what? Perhaps there would be not much of anything, since we are biological beings, a sophisticated collection of cells. There would simply be nothing at all.

Yet cells are in fact a small part of connective tissue's overall contribution to human structure. It is the extracellular material that gives the various connective tissues their characteristic shape, tensile strength and texture. Without its cells, connective tissue would still provide the body with a degree of shape, a range of tissue textures and, perhaps, even a semblance of our 'cells-included' appearance. Connective tissue is mostly about its non-cellular characteristics. Cars – the living things of the highway – drive over bridges and through tunnels, the non-living structures of the highway itself. Take away the cars and the highway remains.

To understand connective tissue fascia is, in part, to appreciate the ECM, a substance that is, by definition, non-cellular in nature and yet, curiously, central to the function of all cells throughout the body.

Extracellular matrix

The ECM of connective tissue consists of fibers and ground substance. There are three types of fibers: collagen, elastin and reticulin. Collagen is the most tensile of the three and is found in fascia, bones, tendons and ligaments. Elastin is less tensile but, as its name suggests, has more elastic qualities. It is found primarily in the lining of the arteries. Reticulin, the least tensile and most elastic of the three, is found in the supporting structures surrounding the glands and lymph nodes. The ground substance is a viscous, gel-like substance in which the cells and fibers lie. The ground substance acts as a mechanical barrier to foreign matter and is a medium for the diffusion of nutrients and waste products. Of particular interest is the fact that it maintains the critical distance between adjacent collagen fibers. This distance allows for some of the extensibility of fascia by reducing the number of microadhesions that can occur between collagen fibers.

The primary components of the ground substance are glycosaminoglycans – sometimes called mucopolysaccharides – and water. There are two types of glycosaminoglycans: sulfated and non-sulfated. The non-sulfated group acts to bind water while the sulfated types give cohesiveness to the fascia. This capacity for binding water is an important aspect of the physiology of fascial disorganization, dehydration and restriction, all of which are discussed later.

Connective tissue types

The strength of connective tissue is determined by the arrangement of the fibers and the viscosity of the ECM. Most histologic sources classify ordinary connective tissue into dense and loose types. These categories are both then divided again, into regular and irregular types.

Dense regular connective tissue, which includes tendons and ligaments, is characterized by a dense parallel arrangement of collagen fibers. The parallel arrangement of the fibers and a high proportion of fibers to ground substance means the tissue is not particularly extensible. Rather, it is extremely

compact so the vascular supply is limited, which accounts for the increased healing time after trauma.

Dense irregular connective tissue includes aponeuroses, joint capsules, periosteum, dermis of the skin and fascial sheaths under high loads of mechanical stress. The fibers are arranged in a multidirectional manner which enables resistance in three dimensions to various forces and stress. The relative amount of ground substance is higher.

Loose irregular connective tissue includes superficial and deep fasciae, nerve and muscle sheaths and the endomysium which holds the individual muscle fibers together. It is characterized by a sparse, multidirectional framework of collagen and elastin with more ground substance per unit area and higher vascularity than the other types (Fig. 2.1).

Thixotropy

Many writers have proposed that connective tissue fascia can be transformed from a gel (thickened) state to a sol (liquid) state by the application of energy.[1,2] This energy isn't mystical or amorphous. In the context of a touch-based therapy such as direct technique MFR, it is accurately defined as the shearing force that is generated within the soft tissue by the application of pressure (force) with direction via hands, knuckles and elbows.

If you've ever stirred a can of paint then you've seen and felt how the consistency of the paint is changed as the shearing force – the paint stick – moves through the liquid. Paint that was thick and gluey becomes more fluid and uniform in texture. The thick gel state gives way to a more liquid sol state. Furthermore, the paint stays in a transformed state for some time after the shearing force is removed. When we apply direct myofascial techniques to restricted tissue we could be seen as the paint stick, stirring (slowly) the fascial can of paint. This transformative process, of gel to sol, is referred to as *thixotropy*.

Effects of immobility

With immobility, changes in the ground substance occur, including losses of glycosaminoglycans and water.[3] Since the non-sulfated glycosaminoglycans bind water, the loss of water is easy to explain. Lubrication between the collagen fibers is

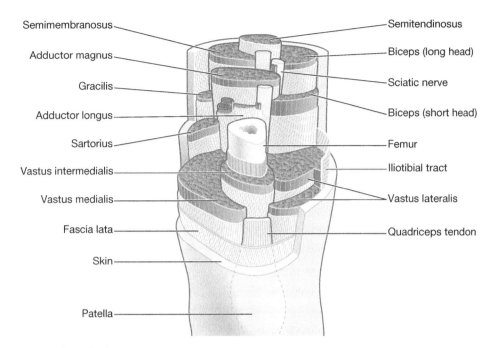

Figure 2.1 Layers of myofasciae.

maintained by the ground substance. When this critical interfiber distance is not maintained, due to lowered amounts of water and glycosaminoglycans, adjacent collagen fibers move closer together and microadhesions start to occur. As movement helps orient newly synthesized collagen, new collagen in immobilized (stiff) fascia will be laid down in a haphazard manner. Additional binding occurs as the new and randomly arranged collagen forms microadhesions to existing fibers.

The early bonding of these crosslinks consists primarily of weak hydrogen bonds. The hydrogen bonds are eventually replaced by much stronger covalent bonds which require more energy to be broken.

This stiffness, with its attendant physiologic changes, can be seen as the can of paint starting to thicken, from a sol to a gel.

Furthermore, these mechanical and viscous changes at a micro level are responsible for distortions in the quality of movement of joints at a macro level.

A restricted joint often exhibits a diminished range of motion as well as a significant reduction in the quality of graded movement. Even a joint moving within acceptable ranges of motion may exhibit a premature increase in binding when approaching that end range. Active testing across multiple planes of motion (real-world movement) will reveal some zones that are grabbing, stiff and boggy as the fascial strains appear to prevent utilization of the full movement potential. Passive range of motion reveals early binding approaching end range and irregular soft tissue tensions. The constant 'stirring' of the fascia that occurs as a joint moves freely within the parameters of its anatomic design is further diminished or lost.

Stiffness, it seems fair to say, leads in time to more stiffness.

Scar tissue

The histology and biomechanics of scar tissue differ from those of non-traumatized connective tissue. As they are frequently encountered, scars deserve additional examination.

Scar formation consists of four major phases.

1. The inflammatory phase begins immediately after the insult to the tissue, followed a short time later by clotting. Soon after that there is an influx of macrophages and histiocytes. They are involved in debriding the area, which promotes a clean

environment for healing. This inflammatory stage lasts from 24 to 48 hours. Immobility is important at this stage to prevent further damage.

2. Granulation, the second stage, involves an increased vascularity of the tissue. Debris is transported away from the area, while nutrients are transported to it. The length of this granulation phase varies depending on the type of connective tissue involved and the extent of the insult.

3. The third phase of scar formation is the fibroblastic phase. There is a proliferation of fibroblasts and an increase in their activity. The rate of collagen and ground substance formation increases. Collagen is laid down haphazardly during this phase which lasts from 3 to 8 weeks.

4. In the maturation phase collagen production is still accelerated. However, there is an overall shrinking, solidifying and consolidation of the collagen. In this phase collagen is strong enough to endure some therapeutic stress without incurring further damage. This is a phase when the deformative properties of connective tissue fascia can be best exploited by applying direct technique myofascial release to help orient the newly created fibers.

Left unchecked and untreated, the localized 'haystacking' of collagen and the contraction of the tissue will combine to permanently reduce local extensibility. Prolonged periods of immobility, which often occur in an orthopedic situation, exacerbate this condition. Ground substance is lost, with associated increases in intermolecular adhesions. Macroadhesions form between the scar tissue and the surrounding healthy tissue. This limits the extensibility of large sections of tissue which in turn initiates compensatory patterns of hypo- and hypermobile tissue throughout the entire structure. These can lead to areas of stiffness and pain developing in areas quite distant from the initial scar formation.

Scar tissue is also associated with an undesirable increase in the afferent signals to the central nervous system. This neurologic aspect of scar tissue is discussed later.

ALTERNATIVE THEORIES FOR MYOFASCIAL RELEASE

The viscoelastic explanation for the palpable changes associated with fascial release enjoys widespread

support.[1,2,4-6] It has become, in a sense, a classic theory, adopted by many schools of manual therapy. According to this theory, fascia responds to the mechanical interventions of therapy in three related ways.

1. The ground substance changes its volume and consistency.
2. The crosslinkages between the fibers are broken.
3. The interfiber distance is increased so that fiber affinity is reduced, resulting in increased extensibility in the tissue.

Others dispute the capacity of fascia to undergo such rapid change through mechanical deformation alone.[7,8] The arguments advanced against the thixotropy, gel–sol model include the absence of sufficient force delivered over a long enough period of time to produce that type of change. One study showed that moderate elongation of the iliotibial band must be sustained for 1 hour or more for the deformation to be permanent.[7] More forceful methods delivered over a significantly shorter period of time would result in significant tearing and inflammation. In addition, even these deformations appear to require a force far greater than even the largest manual therapist could deliver.[7]

The proponents of these arguments against the thixotropy explanation consider other factors more important to explain the rapid changes that can be felt under the hands of a therapist during the delivery of myofascial release. Rarely do these contacts approach even 2 minutes, let alone 1 hour. What accounts for these quick responses in myofascial extensibility and pliancy? Explanations that go beyond the thixotropy model are based on an exploration of what I will call neurofascial physiology. These important theories are reviewed in conjunction with the following sections on the autonomic nervous system, neuromotor system and the intrafascial mechanoreceptors.

Autonomic nervous system

Some of the mechanical and viscid effects of myofascial release have already been highlighted. In addition, somatovisceral and somatoparasympathetic reflexes are activated by direct technique myofascial release. These responses in the autonomic nervous system (ANS) are at the heart of the changes that occur in response to direct technique MFR. Research supports this neurofascial dynamic as being an important aspect of the types of release observed during MFR.[9] Practitioners of other manual therapies also see change in the ANS as being a significant component of their method.[1,7,10,11]

The ANS has two divisions, the sympathetic (SNS) and the parasympathetic (PNS). Parasympathetic outflow is largely through the vagus nerve. The PNS regulates the functions required for long-term survival and is in charge of rest, rebuilding and rehabilitation. Increasingly, it is seen as having a direct effect on muscle tone as well as the more 'vegetative' functions it has traditionally been associated with.

The SNS, at its most extreme, is responsible for the famous fight or flight reflex. It takes care of crises, be they real threats to physical well-being (the local bus headed for you at the crosswalk) or imagined (the overwhelming physiologic responses associated with stage fright or the total collapse in value of a highly leveraged stock portfolio). It also plays a role in the regulation of muscle tone. As can easily be imagined with the fight–flight system, activation of the SNS leads to increases in muscle tone which would obviously facilitate the ability to fight and flee. Equally as obvious is the undesirable state of sustained high SNS tone. A range of serious disorders is associated with such an arousal state.

The two branches usually work as antagonists. Gellhorn proposed a law of reciprocal inhibition that describes a dynamic whereby the excitation of one branch leads to the inhibition of the other.[12] He also proposed that long-term tuning of the ANS is possible. In this situation one of the branches dominates the other in such a way that the reciprocal inhibition becomes fixed and unchanging.[13]

The balance between these two components of the ANS is central to the self-regulating processes of the body known as *homeostasis*. One definition of stasis proposes it is a state of inactivity caused by opposing equal forces while another is that it is a stagnation in the flow of any of the fluids in a body. In the end, neither definition conveys the need for a flexible and adaptive nervous system that can constantly fine-tune the well-being of the organism. A prolonged state of imbalance or stasis, associated with Gellhorn's tuning, is detrimental to health across a broad spectrum of core bodily processes. The term 'homeokinesis' is probably

more suited to describing a healthy relationship between the two branches of the ANS.[14] Ideally there is a play between the two throughout the day, a healthy range of flexible sinusoidal movement from one branch into another (Fig. 2.2).

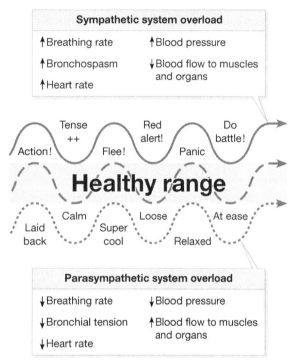

Figure 2.2 Autonomic nervous system showing healthy range and out-of-range problems. Gellhorn's tuning takes place when the ANS stays fixed in one of the overload zones. Generally, with MFR pain and stiffness this is in the extreme of the SNS range (after Bradley,[16] with permission).

Various authors have attributed the success of manual therapies to the restoration of ANS modulations back into the healthy range. Upledger sees the restoration of autonomic flexibility as one of the primary benefits of craniosacral therapy.[10] Dr Ida Rolf held a similar view about the benefits of Rolfing®.[5] When describing the formation of the cranial rhythmic impulse (CRI), McPartland & Mein proposed that:

... if our hypothesis and findings from entrainment studies are true, then the common denominator and underlying mechanism generating CRI is the balance between the sympathetic and parasympathetic nervous systems. If there is autonomic nervous system balance then

the body's rhythms harmonize into a strong, coordinated, sinusoidally fluctuating entrainment frequency, palpated by the practitioner as a strong healthy CRI. To wit, health as assessed by CRI becomes dependent on sympathovagal balance.[15]

The importance of the ANS for health should not be underestimated. Consider that all cells have sympathetic innervation. The impact of a chronically aroused SNS, coupled with the outflow of the associated stress hormones, will therefore be profound. It can stall healing, generate hypertension, contribute to the formation of facilitated segments, impair metabolism via endocrine imbalance and ultimately all homeostatic (kinetic) mechanisms. Chronic hyperventilation, with an associated loss of oxygen to the brain, resulting in multiple diminished functions, is another serious consequence.[16]

Considering the frequency of asthma, hypertension, glaucoma, ulcer disease, and abnormalities of sweating, temperature, cardiac rhythm, respiration, sexual, bowel and bladder function, it is amazing that the autonomic nervous system gets essentially no direct treatment.[11]

This observation accurately describes the scope of the health problems associated with the ANS. However, the assertion that there is little direct treatment of the ANS is not accurate. Direct technique MFR provides that treatment.

Studies have found that certain forms of tactile stimulation produce predictable changes in the ANS. Deep slow pressure into the skeletal muscle of cats produces a decrease in blood pressure (under control of the ANS).[17] More germane to a practitioner of direct technique MFR are studies into the relationship of tactile stimulation and ANS responses in humans. Using a vagal tone monitor to assess the activity of the vagus nerve, researchers have demonstrated that the PNS was stimulated by direct technique MFR to the sacrum and low back.[18,19] These studies indicate that soft tissue pelvic manipulation is useful for certain types of low back dysfunction, as well as musculoskeletal disorders associated with autonomic stress and imbalance.

From my own clinical practice, I observe that deep calming of the type associated with increased PNS activity often occurs during a treatment using direct technique MFR. The signs of this include:

- borborygmus (bowel sounds – gurgling, pinging and the like)
- hypnogogia (the dreamy fluid state between waking and sleeping)
- muscle twitching
- deep abdominal jerks and twitches
- fasciculation (skin ripples)
- increased salivation (sometimes drooling)
- full body lowering of muscle tone
- reduced respiratory rate
- full sleep, although this is nowhere near as common as hypnogogia
- lowered heart rate.

Just as important, of course, are the subjective experiences of the client. These include feeling at peace, languid, centered, calm with less rigid thinking and sometimes dream images. This psychosomatic state and its associated dream images are generally pleasant. The sense of the passing of time also alters, usually toward a more timeless, fluid state. These changes are all a function of increased PNS activity.

However, this is not always the case. The opposite effect is sometimes witnessed. Sweating, rapid pulse, increased breathing rate, dry mouth and full body increases in muscle tone can occur. The subjective reports are of irritability, agitation, anger, fear and disordered thinking which are a function of activation of the SNS. These unpleasant sensations are not long lasting. Rather, they appear to be part of an internal psychosomatic integration cycle that is necessary for the restoration of ANS flexibility and homeokinesis.

I definitely favor an increase in the PNS! While spikes in the SNS can occur in manual therapy settings, they should not be provoked through aggressive, invasive approaches. When spikes occur, stop working and allow for the self-regulatory processes of the client to calm them. This is often as simple as waiting for a minute or two at which point the person will report that the effect has passed. Occasionally, more time is needed. I want to emphasize that the goal is to avoid these spikes in SNS activation. Working with direct technique MFR in the mindful, sensitive manner described in this workbook should result in consistent reductions in the chronically aroused SNS – the state associated with musculoskeletal and myofascial pain.

Clearly, the ANS controls, from the top down, a wide range of somatic functions. Appropriate and continuous sensory stimulation from the bottom up, to the brain, is essential for normal brain function. By providing these sensory inputs, direct technique MFR favorably influences the brain and therefore the CNS controls on the ANS. Consider that damage to the sensory cortex is generally more problematic than damage to the motor cortex. Disordered or absent sensory input is catastrophic for the function of the brain itself, as well as the efferent neuromotor system, whereas damage to the motor cortex is often less disintegrative as the underlying sensory afferents are intact. In time, the brain is able to use new regions to formulate motor efferents.

The work of Cottingham and others into the effects of soft tissue manipulation on the ANS is the best explication of these dynamics to date.[18,19] Given the relative ease of measuring the activity of the vagus nerve via a vagal tone monitor, as shown by Cottingham, there could be more research of this kind. Perhaps in the near future more studies will explore these fascinating and important relationships.

Neuromotor controls and the central nervous system

Myofascial release also elicits obvious and predictable responses in neuromotor control. Co-contraction, which results in loss of strength, poor joint stability and fatigue through excessive demands by the muscles for energy, is reduced. There is a subsequent increase in muscle recruitment efficiency. This change can be measured by palpation, functional strength testing and range-of-motion tests. The client's subjective report post release will often focus on freedom of movement, decreased stiffness, lightness and better coordination.

An increase in the quality of movement at the joint nearest the site of the myofascial release will be consistently observed. Quality refers to the establishment of a balanced relationship between the agonists and antagonists. The joint is both free moving and stable at all points of its range of motion. Even brief myofascial release can bring about such changes.

Clearly, the effects of the MFR work extend into the nervous system. How does the neuromotor system get involved with manipulation of the body's connective tissue structures? The most obvious explanation for the observed changes in tonus can be found in the process of reciprocal inhibition. This is a muscle tone process, not the reciprocal inhibition of Gellhorn and his descriptions of the ANS. When a muscle on one side of a joint contracts, the muscles on the opposite side should be inhibited to allow for passive lengthening. Without this dynamic, movement would be impossible as muscles on all sides of a joint might fire at the same time. As shortened muscles are lengthened through MFR, the antagonist muscles are released from a long, weakened and inefficient position. This enables the antagonist to resume a tonus that more adequately stabilizes the joint. The process is accelerated via active client movements which activate the antagonist while the therapist applies MFR to the agonist.

A more comprehensive understanding of MFR and the nervous system can be formed by a review of the relationships between structure and function. The ability to maintain posture, or the gravity response, and all movement requires an integrated interplay between a number of systems: the structural or connective tissue elements, the coordination or muscular-motor system and the perceptual or sensory system.[20]

For example, the joint receptors (sensory) provide information to the nervous system that a joint is stable or not. A balanced, even pressure at the joint sends the signal that the joint is working well. To maintain this type of balanced relationship at the articular surfaces requires a sophisticated level of coordinated muscular work. Smooth concentric contraction of the agonists must match well-graded eccentric contraction of the antagonists. The receptors in ligaments, fascia, tendons and viscera are also involved with sensory feedback to the central nervous system, which in turn develops appropriate, or inappropriate as the case may be, coordination via the motor system.

The efficient, well-ordered firing of muscles is dependent on appropriate sensory information that is processed to generate a normal efferent signal. A feedback loop is developed here. Any disruptions to the sensory signals, from the joints, ligaments, tendons or muscle spindles, can alter the tone of muscles as well as their firing order. Disruptions to these signals occur for a variety of reasons – trauma, asymmetrical postural demands on the joints, excessive physical demands, fluid pressure increase, visceral strain, psychomotor posturing, and so on. The list is long but the effect is the same: the bombardment of the CNS with multiple sensory signals from distressed viscera, muscles and joints leads to changes in the neuromotor system. These excessive signals are distributed throughout the CNS and are not confined to one spinal segment – cortex, brainstem and nearby spinal segments will also be affected. The underlying and largely unconscious muscle tone that is essential for maintaining the anti-gravity response – posture – is governed by the gamma motor system. This sustained background tone is referred to as the gamma bias. When the CNS is bombarded with continuous and excessive sensory input, the gamma bias, or sustained efferent outflow, often becomes what is called the gamma gain. Muscle spindles, each contained in their own connective tissue sheaths, become sensitized so that the reflex contraction of a stretched muscle increases. A muscle in this condition resists lengthening. If the gamma gain is sufficiently high the sensitized spindle may force a contraction even when the muscle is shorter than its resting length. Of course, such a condition is extremely dysfunctional with severe negative effects on joint range and stability. This in turn generates more noxious sensory stimuli into the nervous system.

Left unchecked, these sensorimotor disturbances become long-term changes in the structural, connective tissue system. Fascia shortens and thickens in an attempt to provide support where the imbalanced relationship between hypertonic and hypotonic muscles cannot. Further disruptions to the normal physiology of fasciae occur as the full range of movement at the joints and in the muscles is lost, preventing the orientation of newly created collagen fibers.[21] Without appropriate orienting forces, the fibers tend to cluster and thicken. The longer these processes of tightening, compression and misalignment go uninterrupted, the more noxious afferent stimuli there are. These stimuli are not coming solely from the proprioceptors in the muscles, the spindles, but from many types of sensory endings that exist in the connective tissue network. These are elaborated on in the section on intrafascial mechanoreceptors below. Whatever its origins, the cycle is self-perpetuating: constriction, left uninterrupted, leads to more and more serious constriction.

Direct technique MFR as described in this book works into the myofasciae and other connective

tissue types. The thixotropy theory proposes that the action of this mechanical pressure is sufficient to elongate and decompress restricted fascia. Taken alone, this may not be a viable explanation. However, that same deep, slow and directed pressure is also

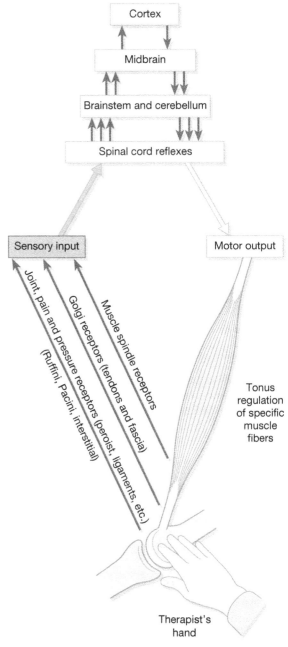

Figure 2.3 The practitioner's touch alters the signals being sent to the CNS. Such disruption to the habitual patterns of the nervous system is a central part of direct technique MFR (after Schleip,[7] with permission of the author).

affecting a range of sensory fibers via stimulation of the joint, ligament, muscle and tendon receptors. In Figure 2.3, we see the therapist's hand involved in altering the dynamics of the biofeedback loops outlined above. The noxious stimuli that result in the self-perpetuating pain, compression and dysfunction cycle are replaced with new afferent signals. These, in turn, alter the efferent signals.

For example, changes in tone create a change in joint position, which in turn helps normalize tone. Over the long term these initial and rapid changes in tone, coordination and perception lead to a more appropriate arrangement of collagen fibers within fascia. Contrast this with the more conventional view that this restructuring of the connective tissue happens immediately, as proposed in the thixotropy model.

Intrafascial mechanoreceptors

In the opening section of this chapter, we saw that fascia was part of the large ECM of the body. A theory of fascial release, generally identified as thixotropy, was developed. The release is seen as involving a mechanical stretching of the fibers as well as an associated change in the hydration of the ground substance.

Next I introduced alternative theories of fascia release that included somato-autonomic reflexes. Reflexes require an initiating sensation and that means sensory fibers. As this section will show, they are in fact enormously important to understanding what happens under our hands when we touch someone.

Sensory fibers within the fascia itself have a highly developed capacity to communicate with both the ANS and the CNS.[22] For myofascial therapists seeking to flesh out a theory of why MFR works, these sensory fibers – Ruffini, Pacinian and interstitial – are the El Dorado of neurophysiology.

Within dense regular connective tissue there are two types of mechanoreceptors: the Pacinian/Paciniform corpuscles and the Ruffini bodies.[23] Thus, they occur within myofascia, tendons, aponeuroses and ligaments, the very soft tissues we focus on in direct technique MFR. These are in addition to the sensory fibers that lie within the muscle – spindles and some of the Golgi tendon organs (GTOs). The role of the GTOs in inhibiting

tone is well documented although it is now thought that they discharge only when muscles actively contract. They respond to changes in force, not length. Direct technique MFR applied to a muscle that is actively contracting against resistance, usually eccentrically, increases the discharge from the GTOs and elicits inhibition of any further tensioning in that muscle.

The Pacinian corpuscles are stimulated by high-velocity, low-amplitude (HVLA) thrust manipulations, as well as vibratory techniques while the Ruffini bodies respond to slow and deep melting techniques.[7] Furthermore, the stimulation of the Ruffini bodies is linked to a reduction in the activity of the SNS. This certainly helps in understanding the effects of soft tissue manipulation on the ANS that were described earlier where both local and systemic changes in that system occur.

Gamma neurons can be inhibited by supraspinal structures. The medial reticular formation plays a role in this inhibition. As we saw in Figure 2.3, the various sensory fibers found in fascia make connections to the brainstem and above. They are not directly involved in the local myotactic reflex arc taking place at the spinal segment. It is likely that these various sensory fibers are involved in carrying information to the CNS that reestablishes inhibition of gamma gain from the top down. This would account for the fact that many rapid changes in tone take place when applying direct technique MFR to tissue that is completely devoid of muscle fibers. For example, a deep slow MFR technique applied to the calcaneus will elicit a predictable change in range of motion at the ankle, with obvious reductions in gastrocnemius tone with an increase in its resting length. Additionally, coordination and stability will improve even though no deliberate attempt is made to balance the action of agonists and antagonists. The spindles have not been directly treated. Although the processes are not clear, I propose that these changes are a function of sensory inputs ascending to supraspinal levels and influencing the formation of inhibition.

The third group of nerves is the interstitial muscle receptors. Researchers have identified their involvement in the fine tuning of the blood flow. This also points to a direct connection to the ANS. Sakada's study of the periosteum of the mandible shows slow and rapid responding receptors. The slow receptors sense pressure and pain, as well as low-frequency vibration. The rapid-response receptors are involved in sensing pressure and pain but also much higher frequency vibration, up to 500 Hz.[22]

The interstitial fibers have been shown to have control over plasma extravasation.[24] This refers to the extrusion of plasma from blood vessels into the interstitial fluid matrix. Now we see a nervous system component to the gel–sol model described earlier. When certain forms of stimulation are present, of the kind provided by an MFR practitioner, the interstitial fibers signal the blood vessels to increase the renewal speed of the ground substance. Hydration may occur but it is initiated through sensory fibers rather than mechanical force alone.

An increase in the quantity of ground substance helps maintain the interfiber distance and lubricates the space between the fibers. This is fascial cohesiveness – the affinity of fibers that drives them to bind with their neighbors is balanced via an appropriate volume of ground substance. As the neuromotor system is released from dysfunction via MFR, fascia is stressed via appropriate and orderly movement. Collagen will be laid down according to the general direction of the stress. Movement forces fibers into extensibility and this prevents the clumping of collagen fibers. A combination of increased levels of ground substance with more orderly arrangements of fibers means fewer crosslinks and increased extensibility.

Once the intrafascial mechanoreceptors are included in the discussion, a bigger, fuller picture emerges, of therapist-induced forces acting to trigger complex neurologic reflexes that quickly alter the tonus of both the ANS and the CNS.[7,13,18,19] In turn these changes have numerous direct and indirect effects on the ground substance and fascial cohesiveness in general.

AND THERE'S MORE ...

Smooth muscle cells have been found in the fascia cruris (fascia of lower leg). Using electron photomicroscopy, two researchers observed not only widespread existence of the intrafascial nerve fibers mentioned above but also, unexpectedly, smooth muscle cells.[25] While we are already in a kind of neurofascial El Dorado, this discovery amounts to a jackpot in the exploration of the relationship between fascia and the nervous system. With smooth muscle cells being under the control of the ANS, it seems likely that neural-regulated tensioning occurs within fascia. This fascial tonus is controlled via the state of the ANS, separate but related to the much stronger tonus regulation of muscles via the neuromuscular system. What the purpose of this 'pretensioning' might be is not clear. While this is debated, it seems possible to conclude that an ANS tuned toward the SNS branch might exert an overtensioning effect on the fascia. MFR has been shown to reduce the severity of this tuning and increase the activity of the vagus nerve. It could well be that part of the release and lengthening the client and therapist both feel during the application of MFR is a tension release in the intrafascial smooth muscle cells.

PIEZOELECTRIC EFFECT

A lesser developed theory for the kind of fascial deformation we are seeking to understand is the piezoelectric effect. Piezo (pressure) electricity refers to the generation of an electrical charge when a crystal is compressed. Connective tissue may act as a liquid crystal. At least one author has proposed that the application of the therapist's pressure increases the electrical charge within the tissue.[26] This, in turn, stimulates the fibroblasts to increase the secretion of collagen fibers in that local area.

A number of problems exist with this theory. First and foremost, the secretion of fibers could not occur so rapidly that a therapist would sense that production. Also, the secretion of fibers across any timespan would not account for the rapid changes in tissue texture that are palpated during direct technique MFR. Nor would the increased production of fibers necessarily be a desirable state for the body.

However, activation of the piezoelectric effect may provide the necessary charge for the stimulation of the sensory branch of the interstitial fibers. In turn, these have control over plasma extravasation, which is associated with ground substance hydration/dehydration. Sakada's research shows interstitial fibers as being sensitive to low- and high-frequency vibrations. Perhaps it is here, at the level of the interstitial fibers, that the piezoelectric effect is playing a part in fascial structure and function.

PSYCHOSOCIAL FACTORS

Manual therapy often describes the body as if there is, in fact, a pure body that exists separately from social and cultural contexts. I write this book in Australia as if there is a universal body to be discussed and engaged with. It's a complex dilemma. Certainly, our biological body can be understood in terms of a semi-universal anatomy and physiology. To a great extent, a muscle spindle is a muscle spindle in whatever body it might be found, with a predictable relationship to the central nervous system and muscle tone.

However, what of the way we think about and shape our bodies in other contexts? How could any one author write a book that speaks to the multitude of social settings that shape the self-image of their inhabitants? A woman in Somalia? A teenage boy in central China? An elderly Afghan refugee incarcerated indefinitely in an Australian detention center? A child with cerebral palsy in South Texas? What is the 'self-image' body in these contexts? What is the meaning of touch therapies in the social context in which they are delivered? As numerous social constructivists have proposed when warning about the blinders put on when adopting a purely biological determinism, 'The impact of any biological feature depends in every instance on how that biological feature interacts with the environment'.[27]

This is the realm of the psychosomatic body and, to coin a phrase, the 'sociosomatic' body as well. Numerous authors in the social sciences have of course articulated, from a variety of perspectives, the view that self-image forms in the context of cultural, social and psychological environments. That self-image can, to a great extent, shape many of the processes at work in the biological landscape. Changes made through direct technique MFR could be looked at, although they are not in this book, simply in terms of the anatomic, physiologic and kinesiologic effects described so far. Desirable changes in those three alone would certainly be enough to make direct technique MFR a powerful therapy.

Still, when manual therapy techniques are described and the rationale for using them is elaborated, it can sound like we're talking about simply tuning a soft machine. A form of biological reductionism starts to creep in: all we are is an assemblage of fluid-filled bags moved from one place to another by contractile fibers that are instructed from the

nervous system. Of course, this is a convenient way to analyze and understand certain parts of the whole person. With hard science on their side, these descriptions then sound reassuringly final and conclusive. But what happens in social and cultural contexts when a person moves from a compressed, fatigued and painful state into one that is more at ease and expressive? An example of this non-linear systems thinking is shown in Figure 2.4 where a state of thoracic flexion and tightness is seen as existing in relationship with a number of other aspects of a person.

Are there changes that include, but go beyond, the biological? The observation has been made by many somatic therapists that release from chronic tightness can influence both the psychosomatic and sociosomatic body. The non-linear approach can be developed even further than in Figure 2.4, to include a wide range of relationships that occur between biological, psychologic and sociologic factors (Fig. 2.5). And the opposite is also true. These same psychosocial factors may contribute to the development of disruptions to the normal function of the neuromyofascial net. The shift in thinking is from cause and effect to non-linear interdependencies. Using this dynamic model makes the discussion on what happens in MFR a much more complex one.

The famous Whitehall studies show that the most significant factors for general health are not fitness, diet, genetics or whatever – they are social rank and socio-economic status.[28] In these studies a steep inverse relationship was found between social class and morbidity from a wide range of diseases. A similar relationship was seen between

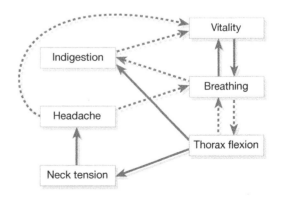

Figure 2.4 Viewing the effects of direct technique MFR from a systems perspective, rather than a linear cause and effect model (from Schleip,[7] with permission of the author).

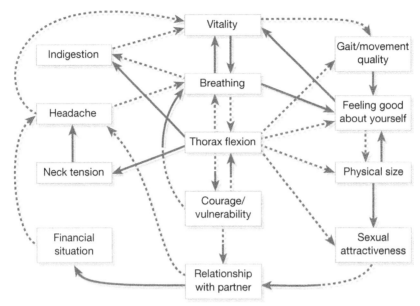

Figure 2.5 An expanded version of these complex interdependencies that includes psychosocial and psychological factors (from Schleip,[7] with permission of the author).

self-observed social status and sick days taken. This finding alone does not prove any direct causal relationship between psychosocial factors and myofascial, or neurofascial, restrictions. Nor is it intended to do so. It becomes of even more interest, though, when other related findings are included. For example, Sapolsky's famous study of baboons showed that a lack of social control leads to high stress as measured by cortisol and adrenaline (epinephrine) levels. Furthermore, his ongoing studies at Stanford University, building on the work of Syles, show that sustained stress can damage the hippocampus, a region of the brain central to learning and memory. His work has identified glucocorticoids, a class of steroids secreted from the adrenal gland during stress, as critical to such neurotoxicity.[29]

As for the psychosocial influences of consumerism and affluence in many Western countries, the same author writes, 'We live well enough to have the luxury to get ourselves sick with purely social, psychological stress'.[30] In other words, we do not need an external pathogen or a collision with a brick wall to introduce serious disturbance into our being. Our self-image, formed in relation to our perceived social standing, can be enough to steer us toward neurophysiological imbalance.

If lack of social control leads to high levels of stress, then understanding the dynamics of power

relations within cultural and social contexts might be just as important in responding to chronic myofascial restriction as a good set of manual therapy techniques. Developing social supports and networks that enable a greater level of personal satisfaction might be a central part of successful outcomes in somatic therapy. Mentoring programs and, for those with more income, personal coaches could be important pieces of the puzzle for people moving away from disabling patterns of constriction! Fostering relationships that nurture is important, as is identifying ones that do not. Education can lead to feelings of control and participation. Social control leads to a change in physiology. The term 'preventive medicine' takes on a new and challenging meaning here!

I started this section by pointing to the difficulty of talking about the 'body' in a universal biological sense. I proposed that self-image arises in social and cultural contexts. My intention was to suggest a fuller, and hopefully more productive, questioning of what might be affected when deep release and repositioning in the support, transport and coordination systems of a person take place. It also enables a more realistic assessment of the limits of our work. These limitations are not always structural but can have their genesis in functions that are intricately tied to social forces.

Box 2.1 Causes of soft tissue dysfunction. The 'something happens' proposal (from Chaitow,[32] with permission).

- Congenital factors (short/long leg, small hemipelvis, short upper extremity, fascial, cranial and other distortions)
- Overuse, misuse and abuse (and disuse) factors (such as injury or inappropriate patterns of use involved in work, sport or regular activities)
- Postural stresses
- Reflexive factors (trigger points, facilitated spinal regions)
- Chronic negative emotional states (anxiety, repressed anger, etc.)
- Nutritional deficits
- Toxic accumulations
- Infection
- Endocrine (hormonal) imbalances

Still, despite this journey into areas outside the biological, I must acknowledge that the breadth of the discussion has been limited. In particular, it focuses on these issues in a Western consumer-capitalist context where personal, individual subjectivities are highly valued, especially within certain socio-economic groups.[31] Certainly, not all cultures, or classes within Western society, place the same emphasis on the formation of these highly individual subjectivities.

A GRAND UNIFYING THEORY?

In examining the causes for disruption to the normal function of the myofascial complex, Chaitow has used the delightfully simple phrase 'something happens'.[32] He then lists the various possible components leading to this disruption (Box 2.1). It is

Box 2.2 The 'everything happens' response to direct technique MFR. The net is cast wide to include the co-emergent relationships that exist between the biological and the social.

- Golgi tendon organs stimulated – tone inhibited.
- Ruffini endings are stretched, resulting in inhibition of overall sympathetic nervous system activity.
- Reductions in SNS activity affect smooth muscle fibers found in fascia = fascial and whole organism decompression. Increased parasympathetic activity enhances whole organism well-being.
- Interstitial receptors are stimulated especially via work on the periosteum, resulting in increased proprioceptive acuity as well as ground substance renewal.
- Muscle spindles are slowly stretched resulting in a lowering of muscle tone.
- Supraspinal inhibition of gamma gain leads to resetting of gamma bias. Gravity response improves.
- Self-defeating cocontraction patterns of movement (agonist and antagonist firing at the same time) are reduced, resulting in heightened energy for creative and expressive movement.
- Mechanical restrictions to breathing are released leading to overall improvement in physiology and balance in CO_2/O_2 ratios in the blood. Further changes in the ANS take place.
- Lymph and all fluid return is improved. Fascial cohesiveness begins to improve.
- Postures of defeat are reduced, allowing for explorations of a new self-image that is oriented in real time and space (here and now, 'take up your space') rather than via inner narrative which is oriented to the there and then ('if only').
- Whole organism decompression leads to new expanded relationship with the environment and more satisfying interactions with it. Self-confidence and esteem are boosted.
- 'It takes two to know one'. The communication taking place in the therapeutic relationship is a springboard to a new formulation of 'self' (for client and therapist). Movement and touch behaviors modeled by the therapist generate new potentials for the client.
- Introduction of neural plasticity (ANS and CNS) leads to better movement that orients new collagen fibers into more supportive and less constrictive arrangements. Refreshing the ground substance creates greater interfiber distance that reduces binding between fibers, long-term changes in fascial cohesiveness now possible.
- Self-regulating function of the body enhanced, resulting in better overall health, especially in all systems regulated by the ANS – basically everything!

possible to use a similarly useful vernacular term and say that the response to direct technique MFR is that 'everything' happens. While this is, of course, not completely true, it does convey the breadth of the witnessed effects. The response is not localized to one system but percolates into many. Non-linear systems theory, with its multitudes of interdependent, co-emergent relationships, makes the 'everything happens' hypothetical model viable, even as it takes the interested reader outside the comfort zone of the more usual cause and effect approach (Box 2.2).

Further reading

Bradley D 1998 *Hyperventilation Syndrome: Breathing Pattern Disorders, 3rd edn.* Tandem Press, Birkenhead
Dinah Bradley is a New Zealand-trained phsyiotherapist who has worked in a wide range of settings. However, her long-time interest has been respiratory therapy, especially the poorly documented syndrome of chronic hyperventilation. This book is written for the lay person who seeks to understand the range of problems caused by hyperventilation. It contains excellent material on the relationship between the ANS, CO_2, anxiety and other unpleasant physiologic events. It provides sufficient information to inform both the health practitioner seeking more understanding of this surprisingly common problem as well as clients who want tools for self-management. I recommend it as a primer. If the material in here is especially relevant to your practice then I suggest going onto the more substantial and excellent *Multidisciplinary Approaches to Breathing Pattern Disorders* by Chaitow, Bradley and Gilbert (Churchill Livingstone, Edinburgh, 2002).

Chaitow L 1999 *Cranial Manipulation Theory and Practice: Osseous and Soft Tissue Approaches.* Churchill Livingstone, Edinburgh
The text is easy to follow and links the theory to the practical problems of the clinician. The book describes both soft tissue and osseous applications as well as providing guidance on which option to select in different clinical situations. Practical exercises are included to help improve clinical skills. Chaitow does a thorough literature review of recent research into cranial motion and rhythm. In fact, this review is one of the book's most important elements. Chaitow uses the information he gathers to challenge much of the previously unquestioned dogma that some of the principal teachers of cranial manipulation still adhere to. While Chaitow's role as iconoclast might offend

some, most readers will find his frank reevaluation of the main cranial theories to be a breath of fresh air in an area that has for too long been muddied by jargon, dogma and isolationist politics.

Chaitow L, Bradley D, Gilbert C 2002 *Multidisciplinary Approaches to Breathing Pattern Disorders.* Churchill Livingstone, Edinburgh
For many years, decades even, I observed a strong link between breathing patterns that seemed less than ideal and anxiety states. Or to put it another way, high rapid breathing was associated with SNS arousal as well as, generally, hypertonic myofascia. Bradley's first book gave real insight into the physiologic processes accompanying chronic hyperventilation syndrome (CHS). Then this much more complex volume appeared, complete with a variety of manual therapy techniques for addressing the physical restrictions of the rib cage that perpetuate the syndrome. This is a great text. If 12% of the general population suffers with CHS, as Bradley suggests, then that alone is significant. But given the relationship between CHS, the SNS, anxiety and changes in myofascial tone, the percentage of people presenting at a manual therapy clinic is probably much higher. It's worth knowing about!

Cottingham JT 1985 *Healing Through Touch: A History and Review of the Physiological Evidence.* Rolf Institute, Bouder, CO
While somewhat dated now, Cottingham's book offers a perspective on aspects of physiology that have immediate relevance for bodyworkers. His investigation into this area turned up many important research findings that might otherwise have gone unnoticed. His seminal research into the autonomic nervous system makes his contribution to the area of manual therapies a significant one. I've hoped for some time that Cottingham might rework this slender text into an updated and more comprehensive version.

Grossinger R 1995 *Planet Medicine, Vols I & II.* North Atlantic Books, Berkeley, CA
The author, who holds a doctorate in anthropology, with a specialization in medical anthropology, has developed a two-volume work that can easily be described as encyclopedic. For anyone with a desire to understand the real history of medicine and be able to place any healing practice in its historical context, this work is required reading. It's especially strong in the area of somatics. While I do not share all of the author's sensibilities, I consider this to be a well-articulated work and highly recommend it.

Juhan D 1987 *Job's Body: A Handbook for Bodyworkers.* Station Hill Press, New York

The style is extremely approachable yet this text contains a great deal of complex information that is useful to anyone interested in touch therapies. The section on muscle tone is excellent and will satisfy the needs of most bodyworkers. This is basically a foundation text for all bodyworkers.

Rolf IP 1978 *Rolfing: The Integration of Human Structures.* Harper and Row, New York

When it was initially published this book was the first of its kind – an attempt to develop a view of holism that included the relationship of human structure to the gravitational field. For Rolf this was the culmination of decades of research, clinical practice and philosophical thought. She drew on her knowledge of fascia (the subject of her doctoral dissertation) to give her work an impressive depth of understanding. Rolf's writing is characterized by precise use of language (influenced no doubt by her studies in General Semantics) and passion for her ideas about balanced posture. Many of her ideas are now so integrated into bodywork practice and jargon that it's easy to forget how original and unique her line of inquiry was. Few people have articulated so fully an original formulation of what integration means, let alone a set of protocols to consistently achieve it. Rolf is definitely one of them.

Schleip R 2003 *Explorations of the Neuro-myofascial Net.* Journal of Bodywork and Movement Therapies 7(1):11–19

Schleip is a master synthesizer. Working from the perspective of a practicing Rolfer® and Feldenkrais practitioner, he has gathered an impressive array of research that is related to his ongoing passion – what happens when we touch someone in therapy? Why does it work? This article, and another from April of the same year, are some of the best contributions to this understanding that I have seen. Schleip blends the findings of solid research into a wonderful narrative about talking to schools of fish, wet tropical neurofascial jungles and other lively analogies. While there is academic rigor displayed throughout, the lasting impression of these articles is that they are fun to read.

Schultz L, Feitis R 1997 *The Endless Web.* North Atlantic Books, Berkeley, CA

Schultz is a long-time Rolfer® as well as having had a previous career as a professor at a major US medical school. Feitis was a Rolfer® before training as an osteopath and now practices medicine and Rolfing®

in New York. Their combined backgrounds enable an examination of fascial anatomy that blends elements of morphology, cytology and embryology into a holistic viewpoint. This, in combination with the overall ease of style, makes this a delightful read and an original contribution to understanding bodies the way bodyworkers need to. For someone beginning to undertand the anatomy of continuity and connection, this is a great place to start.

www.somatics.de

A valuable online resource with articles galore.

References

1. Rolf IP 1977 Rolfing – the integration of human structures. Harper and Row, New York
2. Juhan D 1987 Job's body. Station Hill Press, New York
3. Akeson WH, Woo S, Amiel D et al 1973 The connective tissue response to immobilization: biomechanical changes in the periarticular connective tissue of the rabbit knee. Clinical Orthopedics 73:356–362
4. Little K 1969 Toward the more effective manipulative management of chronic myofascial strain and stress syndromes. Journal of the American Osteopathic Association 68:675–685
5. Rolf IP 1973 Structural integration: a contribution to the understanding of stress. Confinia Psychiatrica 16:69–79
6. Cantu RI, Grodin AJ 1992 Myofascial manipulation: theory and clinical application. Aspen, Gaithersburg, MD
7. Schleip R 2003 Explorations of the neuro-myofascial net. Journal of Bodywork and Movement Therapies 7(1):11–19
8. Threlkeld AS 1992 The effects of manual therapy on connective tissue. Physical Therapy 72(12):893–901
9. Cottingham J 1985 Healing through touch. Rolf Institute, Boulder, CO
10. Upledger JE, Vredevoogd JD 1983 Craniosacral therapy. Eastland Press, Chicago
11. Lynch M 1997 Foreword. In: Giametteo T, Weisilfish-Giametteo S (eds) Integrative manual therapy for the autonomic nervous system and related disorders. North Atlantic Books, Berkeley, CA
12. Gellhorn E 1957 Autonomic imbalance and the hypothalamus. University of Minnesota Press, Minneapolis, MN
13. Gellhorn E 1967 Principles of autonomic-somatic integrations: physiological basis and psychological

and clinical implications. University of Minnesota Press, Minneapolis, MN

14. Godard H 2003 Presentation to the Conference of Structural Bodyworkers, New Zealand (unpublished)

15. McPartland J, Mein E 1997 Entrainment and the cranial rhythmic impulse. Alternative Therapies in Health and Medicine 3(1):40–44

16. Bradley D 1998 Hyperventilation syndrome. Tandem Press, Birkenhead

17. Johansson B 1962 Circulatory response to stimulation of somatic afferents. Acta Physiologica Scandinavica 62(suppl 198):1–91

18. Cottingham J, Porges S, Lyon T 1988 Effects of soft tissue mobilization (Rolfing pelvic lift) on parasympathetic tone in two age groups. Journal of the American Physical Therapy Association 68(3):352–356

19. Cottingham J, Porges S, Lyon T 1988 Shifts in pelvic inclination angle and parasympathetic tone produced by Rolfing soft tissue manipulation. Journal of the American Physical Therapy Association 68(9):1364–1370

20. Frank K 1995 Tonic function: a gravity response model for Rolfing® structural and movement integration. Self-published. Available online at: www.somatics.de

21. Arem AJ, Madden JW 1976 Effects of stress on healing wounds: intermittent non-cyclical tension. Journal of Surgical Research 20:93–102

22. Sakada S 1983 Physiology of the mechanical senses of the oral structure. Frontiers of Oral Physiology 4:1–32

23. Yahia L, Pigeon P, Des Rosiers E et al 1993 Viscoelastic properties of the human lumbodorsal fascia. Journal of Biomedical Engineering 15(9):425–429

24. Kruger L 1987 Cutaneous sensory system. In: Adelman G (Ed.) Encyclopedia of neuroscience. Birkhauser, Boston, pp 293–294

25. Staubesand J, Li Y 1996 Zum Feinbau der Fascia cruris mit beonderer Berücksichtigung epi- und intrafaszialer Nerven. [Detailed structure of the crural fascia with special consideration of the epi- and intrafascial nerves.] Manuelle Medizin 34:196–200

26. Oschman JL 2000 Energy medicine. Churchill Livingstone, Edinburgh

27. Bem SL 1993 The lens of gender: transforming the debate on sexual inequality. Yale University Press, New Haven, CT

28. Marmot MG, Smith GD, Stansfield S et al 1991 Health inequalities among British civil servants: the Whitehall II study. Lancet 337:1397–1398

29. www.stanford.edu/dept/biology/faculty/ sapolsky.html

30. Sapolsky R 2001 A primate's memoir. Scribner, New York

31. Macdonald M 1995 Representing women. Edward Arnold, London

32. Chaitow L 1999 Cranial manipulation theory and practice. Churchill Livingstone, Edinburgh

Chapter 3
HOW TO DO IT

Put the tissue where it should be and then ask for movement. (Rolf)

Doing direct technique myofascial release well is actually quite straightforward. Getting really good at it takes at least 3–5 years. Let's get started.

- Land on the surface with the chosen tool (see Chapter 5).
- Sink into the soft tissue, at 90° to the surface.
- Contact the first restricted layer. This is the level in the tissue where there is obvious tension that would require effort to overcome.
- Put in a 'line of tension': this is an oblique angle of about 30° to the surface.
- Engage through the line of tension by taking up the slack in the tissue without moving across the surface.
- Finally, move across the surface while staying in touch with the underlying layers.
- Exit gracefully.

MOVEMENT

This is simple enough. But there's more, although this is not about MFR being less simple. In fact, the addition of movement makes the work even more straightforward.

The movement that initiates the restoration of myofascial mobility comes from two sources. The first is the micro-stretching that occurs as the practitioner directs pressure into the fascia, usually on an oblique angle. This action is a type of 'therapeutic stress', applied to transmit energy into the elastic, viscous and sensory components of fascia. It is a way of saying 'hello' to all of them. This is described as taking up a line of tension in the fascia. Although

movement of the practitioner's hands would be visible to an observer, the underlying dynamic in the tissue is more important. The surface movements may even appear to be the same as in deep tissue massage although the intent in MFR is considerably different. Inducing a line of tension in the underlying tissue always precedes movement over the surface. This practitioner-induced movement is directed into the milieu of ground substance, collagen fibers and sensory fibers.

The other movement comes from the client who is directed to make a motion that will influence the treated tissue to lengthen and/or mobilize and release. For example, treating the iliotibial band might involve asking for an anterior and posterior tilt of the pelvis. This additional motion will be experienced by the client as an increase in sensation. For the practitioner, it will be felt as an increase in the counterpressure to the line of tension at the point of contact. By directing the client to mobilize the soft tissue, the amount of therapeutic stress along the line of tension is increased. This is one of the hallmarks of direct technique MFR.

Another useful result of the client-generated movement is that it often encourages motion into areas that have been braced, usually with no conscious intent, for some time. Amongst other dynamics, these adaptations generate a limiting proprioceptive feedback loop. Moving to a new end range and exploring a variety of movements that call on new coordination patterns during fascial manipulation can provide rapid reeducation of these feedback loops. The value of this is hard to overstate. Self-mobilization assists in the reformation of the body's internal sensing processes, the ones that organize movement, balance and the gravity control processes.

Self-mobilization also gives the client a good measure of control in the amount of sensation generated during a release. Depending on how sophisticated the client is, it may be necessary to coach her or him on how to perform the desired movement. It works well to stay away from anatomic and kinesiologic terms when asking for movement. For example, while the client is in side-lying position, ask them to move the tailbone toward the wall behind them. This will induce an anterior tilt, the desired movement. Compare this with asking for an anterior tilt that is initiated by pulling the coccyx out toward the wall. The latter assumes both kinesiologic and anatomic knowledge.

GRAVITY IS THE THERAPIST

Direct technique myofascial release involves the application of your bodyweight through your hands and elbows into the client's body. This does not mean that you should slump or collapse into the contact. Rather, we want to use muscle tone to maintain a low-effort but dynamic posture as we work. This is where we take advantage of the skeletal muscles' gamma bias which provides a muscular tone suitable for stability and activity in the gravitational field. To make use of this tone, explore the sense of dynamically reaching through the point of contact and allowing the bodyweight to join with this motion. Reach through the hand/fist/fingers while maintaining a connection through the feet to the floor. When the whole body participates in this way, gravity flows through the contact.

Proceed at a speed that is determined by the tissues under your touch. 'Listen' to the response that you are calling forth so as to be sure that opening and release occur. If you feel the person contract away from your touch, take this as feedback and be responsive by modifying the speed and/or depth of engagement.

Some of the concerns new practitioners of the technique might have are as follows.

- How much pressure do you use?
  Little. You use gravity by reaching rather than pushing. The beauty of gravity is that its energy is always available.

- How much gravity do you use?
  Just enough to feel you'd have to make an effort and hurt yourself to go further.
- Then what?
  Relax. Let gravity do the work. Sink. Reach. Don't push.
- That's all?
  Then use a deliberate sense of direction with your chosen tool to work through the restriction. First, sink and engage and then move/reach through the tissue.
- Really, that's all?
  Well, in fact there is more to it than that. This book provides ongoing orientation to efficient application of the techniques. As you develop confidence in your touch you'll discover an emerging ability to manipulate and palpate at the same time. As you're learning to get to this skill level, go slowly. After you've reached this skill level, go slowly!

Allow for pauses as you proceed. The deeper you go, the more slowly you'll want to go. Thinking in terms of layers helps here. When I engage a restricted layer I'm not concerned if it is deep or superficial. It's the layer where the first unforced engagement takes place. By working there and not beyond, the sensations will be coherent to the client, satisfying and integrative. On the next contact in that same area, a new, deeper restriction layer might become available. This means that the layers are, in a sense, unwrapped as the person is able to meet the contacts in a coherent and mindful manner.

Listen to the client. Stop means stop, even if we are convinced that this is the release that could ease all their problems!

If they don't verbally say stop but their tissues say it by constricting every time you touch them, you'll find it useful to talk about this rather than trying to 'make the best of it'. Making the observation that they seem to be having a hard time letting go will almost always open up the dynamic between the client and therapist. Talking in a warm and supportive way about what you, the therapist, perceive to be happening can take the charge out of their anxieties. It might provide an important opportunity for the client to talk about fear and trust, both of which can be core issues for a lot of people. Receiving treatments of this kind, where some level of undressing is required, can sometimes be a trauma in itself, even if we make the situation as safe and secure as possible. Of course, modesty must be respected. In my training as a massage therapist 23 years ago, immodesty was the ideal, something that everyone should move, or be forced, toward. I even heard of therapists working in the nude (yes, really and yes, it was in California) as a way, I guess, of breaking down the barriers to full self-expression (at least, this might have been the rationale). No wonder massage has had to work hard to reinvent its image as something other than a hedonistic indulgence of the New Age.

Let's assume that you've modified and tuned your level of touch enough to be sure you're not just being too pushy or unresponsive to what the client is capable of working with. Many reasons beyond basic awkwardness about the first treatment might contribute to this guarding response. The meaning of touch varies greatly from person to person. For some people, 'shrinking back' is a deep-seated and programmed response to touch. It may have its genesis in a variety of psychophysical traumas that can make letting go into bodywork difficult, at least initially.

In the same study by Cottingham et al that showed a positive relationship between pelvic soft tissue procedures and an increase in the activity of the vagus nerve, a group of older males who also received the procedure exhibited the opposite response. When the sacral base was counternutated via a soft tissue traction of the lumbar spine and lumbosacral joint in the supine position, their PNS activity actually decreased. The researchers did not conjecture about the possible reasons for this response.

Biological reasons might include a reduction of autonomic flexibility across a lifetime although this does not account for a reduction in the PNS activity in response to the pelvic lift. Psychosocial reasons might include an association of touch with sexual intimacy, particularly in the region being contacted. This then led to a stress response when it was perceived as occurring in an inappropriate setting.

Whatever the reasons might be, it shows that the attitude to receiving manual therapy is affected by a broad spectrum of psychosocial, psychosexual and biological contexts. Often there is a need for some simple guidance on how to relate to touch of a therapeutic nature; how to let go, how to be receptive. In talking about these or other concerns, you may

sense a shift from the client feeling powerless to talk about their inner experience to becoming more assertive in expressing their needs.

I'm not suggesting that we become psychotherapists in our sessions. Of course, no therapist can reasonably expect to relate in depth to all the aspects that constitute a person. But we can be sensitive to the broad range of experience that our clients bring through the door by exhibiting warmth, empathy and curiosity. We would like, I believe, to continually increase the scope of what we can include in our field of interaction, even if we do not ever overtly counsel or do psychological work. It's really about big pictures oriented to context and process, rather than a focus on content alone.

Before working, spend some time explaining what you are going to do. Point out in a straightforward way that work of this kind is often deep but that it should feel satisfying or useful. Discomfort may even be felt, but it shouldn't be overwhelming to the point where they stop breathing. Neither should the work provoke full-body muscle guarding in an attempt to mediate the sensations. In fact, exploring the boundaries of what constitutes useful sensation can be exhilarating and liberating. Coupled with client movement, direct technique MFR can provide a vehicle for moving, literally, out of years of constriction, compression and pain.

AN ORDERED APPROACH

I have created a guide to the most effective integrative application of the techniques. Some themes recur throughout, especially the guidelines regarding the speed/depth relationship, while others are about how best to approach a specific area. These comments are all designed to assist the practitioner in making the work attractive to many layers of a person. This style of touch gets a person's attention because it is intelligent and coherent, not a search and destroy mission. My observation is that people are remarkably good at integrating themselves if these appropriate inputs – coherent and responsive – are provided and no overt disintegrative forces – aggressive and mechanistic – are applied.

A few general guidelines on how to generate an integrated response are given below.

■ 'Feather' the release into the surrounding tissues. Work at a specific restriction will be followed by attention to the adjoining area. For example, releasing the shoulder via the subscapularis, teres major and pectoralis major could be followed by broad work in the upper and lower arm as well as the neck.

■ Constantly monitor the breath. It's a wonderful barometer of how the organism is responding. Even the most stoical, masochistic person will catch their breath when the work is overwhelming their organic well-being.

■ After working to release the primary, obvious stuck areas, spend time on the antagonists to those muscle groups. This will awaken the nervous system from its slumber and give an obvious and rapid increase in proprioceptive acuity. This leads to better control of the joint through all its range.

■ Get permission to work into painful, guarded areas. This can be verbal or via a curious, non-invasive quality of touch that waits for tissue permission before proceeding. Of the two, the non-verbal is the most reliable. People will say things that are not true in an attempt to please the therapist.

■ Always do some work bilaterally even if the second side is only touched for a short time. There is ongoing debate about the need to always work bilaterally. I do because I find it creates an immediate sensory integration that makes the changes feel coherent rather than bizarre. The sense of walking in circles after a thorough release of one lower extremity can be a good way to show off the effectiveness of MFR. But sending someone out into the world with that degree of proprioceptive imbalance is counterproductive.

■ Use the movements given here, or the ones that you'll make up as you go, to fully involve the person in the work. This enables them to modulate sensation and assists in neural repatterning.

■ Watch for signs of exhaustion from too much input: glazed eyes; reluctance to participate with assisted movements; weakening, tremulous voice; diminishing, rather than increasing, coordination; attitudes of resignation such as jaw clamping and pursed lips. If exhaustion is observed, finish soon.

■ In just about all sessions it's good to use the releases to the suboccipital region, or broad neck work, to make sure the head has a feeling of connection to the rest of the body. The incredible concentration of muscle spindles here means that this site can act as the source of system-wide high tone. This ongoing tonus is possible even after deep and effective release in other areas.

■ Base the amount of work to be done on the internal and external resources available to the client. At one end of the spectrum there are deep-seated disturbances to the whole organism, conditions like fibromyalgia or chronic fatigue, where only a small amount of light direct technique work (five techniques, including feathering, or less in a session of 15 minutes) should be done in the first session. Get feedback at the next session about the outcome and discontinue the direct technique MFR approach if exhaustion, inflammation or pain is produced. More robust people will respond favorably to more input (15 or more in a 1-hour session). Input refers to the number of contacts, not only depth.

■ Allow time in every session for a period of self-awareness in standing and walking before the client leaves. Ask for reports of what they feel and notice. These do not have to be complicated or complex. Simple reports will assist with integration and clarity of state of mind and body. Pay attention, with eye contact and receptive body language and communication encouragers like nodding and appropriate verbal responses. Recent studies strongly support the value of appropriate non-verbal behaviors in the therapeutic setting. Body lean, open versus closed body posture, eye contact, smiling and tone of voice all influence patient satisfaction when interacting with health professionals.[1] These types of contact acknowledge the value of the client's self-sense even if objective tests will also be applied to ascertain the efficacy of a treatment. Be personal and supportive. Give them a chance to verbalize their sensation and awareness.

Many clients go into a deeply relaxed state as a session progresses. You'll have to decide whether or not this dreamy, drifting state is how you want the session to develop. It's certainly desirable when addressing deep-seated autonomic strain that is constricting the entire organism. You may want to focus exclusively on this aspect of restriction in a number of sessions. Perhaps it will be most useful to wait for a sustained rebalancing of the ANS before tackling functional activities and reeducation.

However, if you plan to involve the client in neuromuscular reeducation in the same treatment, you may wish to avoid going too deeply down into a PNS-oriented state. Using more active client movements will orient the session toward function rather than drowsiness. A combination of some myofascial release followed by functional activities that immediately utilize the new potentials can be very effective, especially with children. MFR to the ankles and feet can be supported with work on a balance board. Detailed work on the neck and head can be supported by subsequent suggestions about how to sit and work at a computer terminal. The list is almost endless. The proprioceptive and coordination changes brought about by MFR will enable a deeper, more authentic connection with suggestions about new postural positions. Simplicity of instruction coupled with a strong anchoring of the education in sensation is the key to success.

DEVELOPING A STRATEGY

A useful strategy is to identify the involved section, treat it and then treat the sections above and below it. This approach towards the periphery assists with transmitting strain away from the restricted site.

Broad neck and back work can be included in most sessions. It tends to be calming and generates feelings of well-being (see above). Intensive work on the ribs, especially in the axilla, is not recommended at the conclusion of a session. The rib, psoas and adductor releases can elicit sudden increases in sympathetic activity, with associated feelings of discomfort and irritation. Utilize those releases in the first half of the session. This allows time for the resolution of any autonomic activation.

When clients report, or you observe, sympathetic responses – sweating, increased pulse, systemic feeling of discomfort – allow time for these to settle before proceeding. Most sympathetic spikes resolve themselves in a few minutes. If you want to help resolve this situation, do some back work with the client lying prone. Keep the contact broad and general. Encourage some full breaths, focusing the inhalation and exhalation into the area/s of most discomfort.

Such strong autonomic responses are not common. However, since they do occur, it's best to have a strategy in mind. On a few occasions I've had people who needed 10–20 minutes for this SNS activity to calm down.

A DYNAMIC APPROACH

There is no real difference between structure and function; they are two sides of the same coin. If structure does not tell us something about function, it means we have not looked at it correctly. (A T Still, founder of osteopathy)

The old division between a problem being either a neuromotor control issue or a structural disorder is certainly dissolving. Two decades ago a person with a neurologic disorder might be treated with neurodevelopmental treatment (NDT), proprioceptive neuromuscular facilitation (PNF), Feldenkrais or other neuromotor-oriented approaches. An orthopedic dysfunction would traditionally receive a more structural approach, with joint and soft tissue restrictions, as well as strengthening, being the foci of treatment.

A more inclusive approach is increasingly popular. Therapists tend to draw from a variety of approaches in treating a client, whether the diagnosis is of an orthopedic condition or a neurologic one. Clearly, clients with neurologic disorders also have fascial and joint restrictions which may be secondary to, or predate, the neurologic lesion. However, they are still a hindrance to function.

Direct technique myofascial release will improve a client's ability to incorporate movement reeducation. Changes to functional patterns should only be introduced as the myofascial and nervous systems become sufficiently plastic for their incorporation. Once these two systems are able to support the change, the client can explore new movement suggestions. If premature, the attempt to introduce new functional patterns can create more strain as the client seeks to incorporate movements the body is not ready for. A good, if simple, example of this is the strain we eventually feel if we attempt the outmoded directive, 'stand up straight'. Here we see the classic problem of forced co-contraction in an attempt to control posture or movement. It is exhausting and thus unsustainable.

Even intelligent movement repatterning methods – the mostly excellent Pilates method, for example – can fail due to the person's inability to achieve a sufficient state of neurofascial plasticity to incorporate the suggested stabilization patterns. Direct technique MFR in conjunction with Pilates or other core stabilization endeavors may assist in the development of this underlying plasticity. Movement teachers of all kinds are encouraged to consider it when students are unable to connect with the required contraction sequences.

In the client with orthopedic problems, neuromotor control is also compromised. This may take the form of muscle guarding, reflexive inhibition, posttraumatic sensory amnesia or, often, all of these. As the ongoing work into lumbar and pelvic stability has shown, inefficient neuromotor controls will often contribute to the original injury. These aberrant neural patterns can hinder or even prevent recovery as well as increase the risk of reinjury. Neuromuscular reeducation may augment myofascial release and accelerate the resolution of an orthopedic problem. This book seeks to introduce approaches to treatments that incorporate elements of both.

LESIONS

In the person with a central nervous system lesion, myofascial release can be an important adjunct to function-oriented treatments, although I must point out that the outcomes are highly variable. In general terms, working with myofascia in the manner shown here allows a desirable response in the neuromotor system. Therapy is more likely to assist in the establishment of balance and stability against gravity when the fascia is released from chronic restriction, whether that is mechanical or neurologic in nature. With neurofascial release comes better sequencing of muscle activation and more coordination of the body against gravity.

MFR also helps develop a more normal metabolic function. This is no doubt due to the effect on the ANS and its relationship with the digestive and endocrine systems.

The importance of approaching the body in this way should not be underestimated. I have observed, as have the pediatric therapists I have worked alongside, these changes in decades of work with children with cerebral palsy. There is too much clinical evidence to ignore the value of this approach as an adjunct to the function-based ones that form the basis of pediatric therapy. I have seen direct technique myofascial release accelerate and deepen the work of both sensory integration and NDT. And even without specific integrated functional activities, I have seen an increase in the control of fine and gross motor skills.

Reference

1. Griffith CH, Wilson JF, Langer S et al House staff nonverbal communication skills and standardized patient satisfaction. Journal of General Internal Medicine 2003; 18(3):170–175

Chapter 4

BODYWORK: A CONTEMPLATIVE APPROACH

In bodywork and movement literature, it is frequently stated that defacilitation in the practitioner is necessary for their work to be effective. This is often found in descriptions of approaches to doing good cranial work, although I believe that the same state would be desirable in any bodywork setting. In fact, it may be central to the kind of open communication that makes for meaningful touch therapy. But what, or who, is being defacilitated? How can it be cultivated? How do we go about this 'defacilitation' thing?

Contemplative practices are marriages of meditation with an activity. As such, they are a blend of the calmness that accompanies meditation with movement. Brush-stroke calligraphy, some martial arts and ikebana are diverse examples of activities that have a history of deliberate contemplative intent; they have historical credentials and they're worth examining to find out more about this deliberate cultivation of movement with awareness. However, we could fairly say that all of life offers a potential for contemplative action. An exposition on how to develop this mindful movement points to 'defacilitation' and contemplative practice as being close cousins, if not identical twins. One has a technical moniker, the other a more humanistic one.

One of the hallmarks of these practices is that the state of the practitioner during the activity is as important as the form of the activity. Curiosity about our selves in relation to the form is central to the process. With this attitude of mindfulness comes freshness. Each situation is new. A mechanistic response is less likely when we drink in the refreshing sensation of the relationship between self and the environment that is forming in each moment. Attachments to perfect outcomes seem less relevant when we allow this sense of relationship to develop more fully. This is the open road of non-competitive

action. It is not available, for example, via the ritual hardening that accompanies excellence in sport in which the body is split from the mind to bring it under full control. Imperfection is not allowed in this scenario, curiosity is irrelevant. The only useful outcome is victory.

As many of us have already discovered, bodywork is an excellent place to deepen the contemplative approach. For somatic therapists their work is already that – a situation where the rush of a time-oriented world is replaced by feelings of timelessness, openness and increased awareness. A wandering mind, adrift in a discursive fantasia, can be reminded to 'come to its senses' and rejoin the bodily moment. We return quite literally to the situation 'at hand'. And for our clients this is felt as a shift in the relationship – the touch is more responsive, curious and friendly. They feel listened to through this type of touch, rather than done to.

One way to explore further this kind of dynamic interchange between perception, intent and action is to begin meditation practice. In the Buddhist tradition there are two related components. The first, *shamatha*, translates from the Sanskrit into tranquility or calm abiding. Bringing attention to an object of meditation, often the breath, helps stabilize the mind and body. Thoughts and emotions – strong psychophysical sensations – are experienced as they arise and allowed to dissolve on the outbreath. They are not repressed or ignored, simply noticed. This is not a soporific state, nor is there an attempt to travel into an altered state of consciousness free from connection with the corporeal world. It is an open and honest experience of the various textures that constitute our being.

The other component, *vipashana*, is a natural outgrowth of *shamatha*. A stable mind and body give birth to insight or clear seeing. The emotions begin to be seen as tendencies, rather than as solid and substantial. As insight develops, the conceptual and emotional patterns become apparent. At the same time, we begin to recognize that our emotions are not some foreign entity that inhabits us but patterns of response that arise when the right stimulus is present. We might even see that Pavlov's dog exists in all of us.

By placing these qualities in the context of a Buddhist exposition of experience, they might seem like attributes of our being that can only be discovered on the meditation mat at the local Zen center or in a cave in Tibet. However, this is not the case. By seeing these attributes or qualities as natural processes related to intention and perception, any situation can offer an opportunity for their exploration.

In bodywork, we have our manual therapy techniques, delivered through bodily action. Clearly, our work is rich with sensation. It is here, right in the realm of the sensations associated with touch, that we look for the development of *shamatha* or calm abiding. It is through bringing sensation into awareness that the practitioner is able to contact the natural process of resting the body and mind. This is 'defacilitation'.

An exercise

While standing at the treatment table, prepare to assume a typical bodily gesture that you might use for the delivery of one of the techniques described in this book. To be most effective, this small exercise is best done without shoes on. Before actually assuming the gesture, create a small gap in the activity, a premovement pause where you are thinking about but not doing the gesture. Now, lift the toes on both feet so that plantar surfaces go into a light stretch. No overstretch – just sensation. Allow the awareness to follow the opening motion in the feet. Continue feeling the opening; the sensation will naturally amplify once the attention is there. Notice other bodily sensations: tonus in the legs, hips and low back will generally reduce; the breathing softens; the shoulders drop without a stern 'Down, stay'. These are possibilities – the key is to notice what is authentic in your experience. Now allow a deliberate connection with the floor to develop with a clear sense of direction – Down. This is completely internal. There is no knee bend, for example. Again, notice the sensations throughout the body and mind.

Generally, there are a number of predictable and obvious shifts in body awareness. There will be a noticeable reduction in the amount of neuromuscular facilitation. The most likely explanation for this is a lowering of tone in the direction-sensitive gamma motor system although an elaboration of the dynamics of this relationship is beyond the intention of this chapter.

This is now the state of calm abiding, generated as a result of simple sensation ('come to your senses') and not, as one might think when Buddhism is mentioned, a complicated esoteric ritual. The object of meditation is the feet or, more particularly, the deliberate sensation of them. The sole of the foot is awoken from the slumber of its predictable tonus and given a sense of direction. The process is sensation rich but sufficiently discrete to allow for exploration, curiosity and discovery.

From calm abiding comes insight. Now contrast this state of body with another, where you resume the gesture that is to be made to perform the technique. What muscles contract first? Are they related to the gesture or part of an unexamined pattern of preparatory movement that has little relevance to the gesture of the contact being made? A common pattern would be to shorten the whole front aspect of the body – rectus abdominis, pectoralis major, SCM – prior to moving towards a contact, even though these contractions would not augment the touch. Often, the lower erectors also fire to lend a sense of support, albeit a false one, to the spine. But again, the actual experience has to be examined.

In general, there will be many preparatory patterns, often with their genesis in a mental picture of how much effort is required to do a certain technique (mostly way too much). This is what we can start to notice. We use the senses, especially the proprioceptive ones (the foot-awakening exercise is about pressure, stretch and direction) to bring us back to calm abiding. From there the process of insight can be developed without effort. This is quite different from trying to learn 'body mechanics' for good, efficient delivery of technique. The intention is to use the appropriate orientation of the body in space to allow the generation of movement that is spontaneously less effortful.

This can be contacted throughout any treatment. It can be explored while seated – excellent for 'defacilitating' the overactive preparatory processes of a cranial practitioner. To develop connection is to first develop sensation. Sensation with direction, to be specific. First we wake up the senses, then we work in a manner that is natural for our body, not overwhelmed by unrealistic and highly conceptual formulations of what effort is needed.

It can be visited any time while we are working. When you start to feel tight and tired when working, it's often related to a loss of sensation and a high amount of facilitation. Rather than trying to talk yourself down, try going into the kind of sensory reorientation process that I have described here. It can also be the hands that explore the sensation of direction-specific, high sensation awareness; it can be both hands and feet simultaneously. This leads to a happy feeling in both girdles!

Seeing that overfacilitation is part of a pattern, rather than a solid entity that defines our selfhood, enables us to drop the pressure of maintaining it. The stimulus to maintain it can be strong and woven right through the fabric of our being. Self-image issues underlie many of these false formulations.

An example

Jane, a slightly built woman with small hands who has a full practice with clients who love the quality of her touch, attends a workshop and observes a tall, large-boned woman presenting some techniques for mobilizing the bones of the foot. The work is presented as highly physical. Furthermore, the presenter is very competent, with a well-developed sense of humor. Her manual therapy skills impress Jane. So too does her style, which is outgoing, charismatic and engaging. The picture she carries in her mind of how to achieve the same results in her own practice includes the highly physical style of the instructor. Prior to the workshop, Jane experienced some shoulder tensions associated with her work but nothing that felt debilitating. Time goes by and Jane notices that her shoulders are tightening as she works, something that has never really happened before. Even her cranial sessions now seem to be leading to tension in the neck and base of the skull.

Fortunately, she reads this chapter on how to use sensory awareness to cultivate defacilitation. She starts to notice that even before she has touched her client's tarsal bones to mobilize them, her body has adopted a highly toned preparatory state. All the big muscles of both girdles are firing, especially the upper trapezius and pectoralis major in the upper girdle and rectus femoris and hamstrings in the lower. The lower spinal erectors pull her lumbar spine into a slight hyperlordosis. Her breath is held, not a lot but enough to create a slight sense of tension throughout the whole rib cage. By exploring sensation and direction, she returns to a state of balanced tone, adjusts her intention as she works to one that matches her structure and starts feeling more at home in her body. She maintains this awareness for several weeks, revisiting her feet and hands as she works. An insight occurs – mobilizing the tarsal bones works best for her with the finesse of a defacilitated state. Her ability to sense change is dramatically increased when the amount of effort is appropriate to the task and her structure.

Our patterns of overpreparation, shifting subjectivities that give birth to a multitude of self-images and inner narratives that may undermine our well-being are not seen as entities or processes that need to be violently uprooted in some way. Curiosity is enough. Then we discover that our self-hood is not so substantial after all and there is relief in this discovery. This kind of embodied awareness and trust in ourselves, or our non-selves might be a better term, is the beginning of compassion or empathy for the bodily situation of others. The two biggest obstacles to open communication, pride and embarrassment, dissolve in the discovery of our own non-facilitated state. When facilitation fades, so too do the strong formulations of self-hood that come from chronic pretensioning in the neuromuscular system. With a lighter sense of self – enlightenment – there is no real personal territory to protect. The various roles we might play – expert technician, omniscient helper, entertainer, victim, iconoclast – might still arise in the play of our lives but we don't have to feel so strongly identified with them.

All this from a few simple and deliberate acts of self-awareness? Perhaps not. The journey to discovery is surely more detailed than this. Still, the goal here has been to point out that the process of doing bodywork is no different from the more formal situations in which one might go about cultivating calm abiding and insight. Life's situations, all of them, provide this opportunity. There is a common thread which has to do with awakening to the sensation of the present and with that comes immediate, spontaneous insight into the causes and conditions that led to the disconnection in the first place. This potential seems to be part of our humanity. It's not added from an external source.

At some point in our training we become technically proficient. Our skills deliver predictable outcomes and then become comfortable, familiar. This is clearly a necessary stage. Gross feelings of incompetence will do a lot to amplify any overworking of the preparatory process. Still, competence and predictability have their dangers as well. The old saying 'Give someone a hammer and the whole world becomes a nail' is a graphic way of illustrating how they can become problematic. The same response is made to what can be quite diverse situations and realities. Authentic communication is established with a willingness to not know, to not bring out the hammer every time a client walks through the door.

Further reading

Maitland J 1996 *Spacious Body.* North Atlantic Press, Berkeley, CA

If issues of ontology, epistemology and phenomenology in the area of somatics are of interest to you then Maitland is required reading. This is a unique work that tackles the thorny philosophical issues surrounding somatic therapy that have largely gone unexamined in our technique-driven world. The author is an advanced Rolfing® instructor, holds a doctorate in philosophy and is a long-time practitioner of Zen. Although it is at times repetitious, this work nevertheless rewards the reader with important insights into the lesser world of somatics and the larger world of life itself. Its relevance to this chapter lies primarily in the exploration of various ways of viewing 'self' and how these can give way to a greater sense of 'no self'.

Chapter 5
TOOLS OF THE TRADE

A MANUAL THERAPIST'S COMMUNICATION MEDIA

Straw polls conducted in my classes reveal that as many as 45% of participants report some peripheral neuropathies involving the fingers, wrist and/or forearm. Since not all participants are massage therapists – around 20% of them come from other manual therapy traditions, especially physiotherapy and osteopathy – it appears that all types of practitioners are at risk.

Massage therapists injure the carpal ligaments via grasping motions with the hand during kneading-type procedures, especially the abductors digiti minimi and pollicis longus as well as the opponens digiti minimi and pollicis, all of which pull on the flexor retinaculum at the wrist. General narrowing and compression of the thoracic outlet due to sustained thoracic and cervical flexion while working is a related problem. Mobilizing physiotherapists also appear to put the thoracic outlet under strain for much the same reason. When asked about the onset of their problems, most practitioners associate the peripheral neuropathies with their work. Clearly, this is not good.

All practitioners need a set of working tools that can serve them well across decades of manual therapy. Insight into structure and function, along with a big bag of manual therapy techniques, is not going to be useful if a practitioner disables themselves via patterns of overuse, strain and subsequent fatigue.

Apart from the obvious benefits to our patients from the use of these techniques, another equally important one is the benefit to the practitioner of doing direct technique MFR . A variety of tools including the fingers, elbows, knuckles, forearms and, less frequently, the thumbs can be employed. As the following photos illustrate, the slowness of the work enables the therapist to pay considerable attention to body use while treating in this manner. In fact, it's possible to explore many aspects of one's own coordination and economical movement while still paying close attention to the client. This results in much better contact and communication.

Developing these various aspects of coordination, stability and appropriate strength takes around 2 years although refinement may continue across a lifetime. While this conditioning takes place, the practitioner will want to shift frequently from one tool to another.

THE FINGERS

Always keep the fingers slightly flexed with the wrists in a neutral position. Keep a slight arch at the MP joints as well as at the carpal tunnel (Fig. 5.1).

Figure 5.1
Correct: the wrists are in neutral and the fingers are in a slightly flexed position.

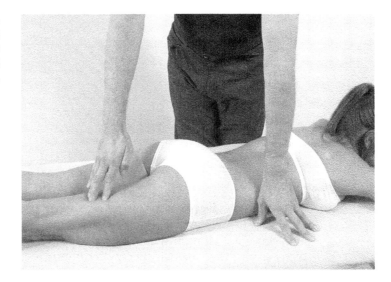

Developing strength and stability in the fingers takes time and practice but unless you are truly 'double jointed', this can be accomplished. Another way to utilize the sensitivity of the fingers without overworking them is to lend stability by working with one hand over the other. This is excellent for sustained contact with minimal effort (Fig. 5.2).

Figure 5.2
Correct: working with one hand on top of the other.

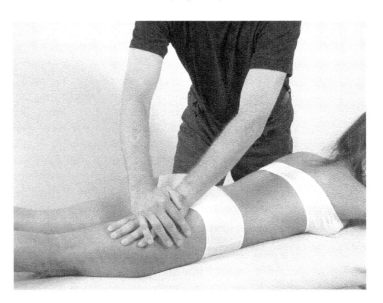

While this conditioning takes place, rest the fingers by making use of the elbows and knuckles. Resting is indicated when the fingers shake, collapse or cannot be prevented from hyperextending (Fig. 5.3).

Figure 5.3
Incorrect: ouch! The wrists
are flexed while the fingers
are hyperextended with
excessive force at the MP
joints.

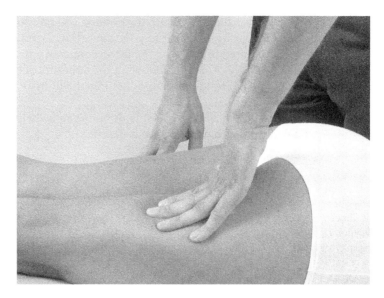

Figure 5.3
Incorrect: ouch! The wrists
are flexed while the fingers
are hyperextended with
excessive force at the MP
joints.

Pain and inflammation in the PIP or DIP joints strongly suggest that earlier signs of strain have been ignored. Even though sensitivity in the elbow and knuckles improves with use, experience shows that the fingers remain the most sensitive tool of all. It's worth spending the time to condition them correctly from the outset.

THE FIST

The fist refers to the use of the four knuckles between the metacarpals and phalanges (MP joints). It is usually a soft fist where the fingers are left extended and folded into the thenar and hyperthenar eminences while the thumb rests lightly on the first finger (Fig. 5.4).

Figure 5.4
Correct: the thumb is
relaxed and the forearm is
pronated sufficiently to
adopt the 'shaking hands'
attitude with the fist.

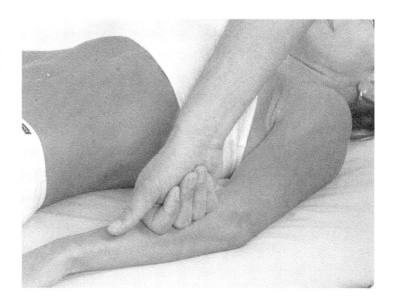

Turn the thumb 'up' into the position you take for shaking hands and you will present your wrist and fist to your contacts in a stable and stress-free manner.

Configured in this way, the fist becomes an amazingly adaptable tool that is quite capable of artfully following the contours of bones, shearing fascial layers or melting through large muscles like the gluteus, all with a wonderful economy of effort (Fig. 5.5).

Bracing the elbow against your body can be helpful at times in which case it will obviously have to be more flexed.

Figure 5.5
Correct: the arm is stable and straight. The weight is able to transmit directly through to the contact site. This is using gravity to bring about release.

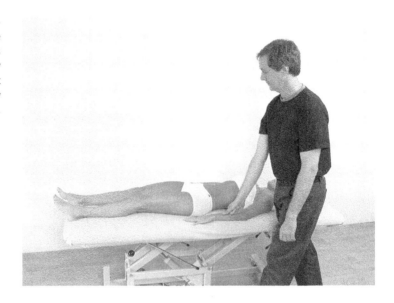

Just as with the fingers, the wrist should be at neutral while the elbow is best kept straight, without taking it into hyperextension (Fig. 5.6).

Figure 5.6
Incorrect: a variation on using the fist that is sometimes used. The weight is going through the carpal bones, placing strain on both the carpal tunnel and the median nerve.

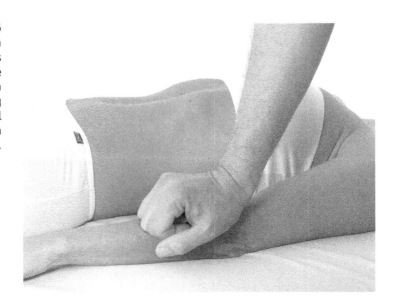

THE ELBOW

These days most therapists are happy to work with their elbows as they've discovered they are excellent tools in a wide range of situations. Our collective carpal ligaments, forearm flexors, median nerves and thoracic outlets no doubt enjoy this development. Although the term 'elbow' is used this is not necessarily accurate as the point of contact can vary. The olecranon process itself is only one possibility. Often, the contact is slightly distal to the olecranon and involves contact through 3–4 cm of the ulna (Fig. 5.7).

Figure 5.7
Correct: the contact is close to the olecranon but not right on it. The fingers are not tense or making a fist.

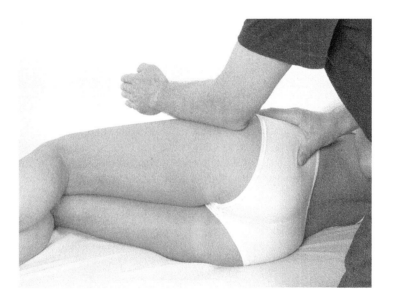

The therapist's skin can become sensitized and even painful during the first few months of working with the elbow. The skin feels like it's being peeled off the bone in a most non-therapeutic manner. Once again, the best response is to shift to other tools and give the overly stressed tissues a rest. Generally, conditioning occurs rapidly and once it's established, there are few complications associated with using the elbow.

Be mindful of the attitude that you bring to working with the elbow. Elbow work need not be synonymous with deep and painful. Use its broad surface area to sink into tight, fibrous tissue with precision. This feels fantastic.

Try to avoid working with extreme internal rotation at the shoulder as, over time, this will cause damage to that joint. Also avoid collapsing into the contact and narrowing the thoracic outlet. The fist should not be clenched (Fig. 5.8).

THE KNUCKLES

The thumbs are vulnerable to injury from overuse and the knuckles – PIPs – can often be used in their place. Like elbows, knuckles can sound like they're simply about intensity of contact. However, there can be a great deal of nuance to their use. The list of situations where they are useful includes the plantar

Figure 5.8
Incorrect: the fist
is clenched and the
shoulder is in full internal
rotation. Too much effort
is being used.

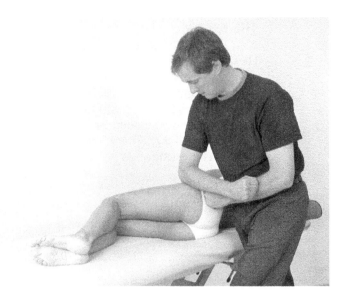

fascia, galea aponeurotica, the retinacula of the ankles and the palmar aspect of the hand. Like the elbow, the contact is rarely right on the points of the joints but spread onto the shafts of the phalanges (Fig. 5.9).

Figure 5.9
Correct: the MP and wrist
joints are at neutral.

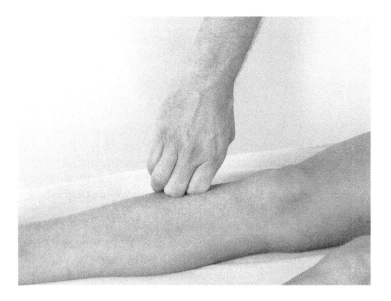

Avoid deviation of the fingers as well as prolonged periods of wrist extension, both of which can lead to sore joints (Fig. 5.10).

THE THUMBS

Of course, sometimes a thumb is just right. However, pay attention to the angles. Hyperextension over a long period of time can render the thumb

Figure 5.10
Incorrect: the fingers are
deviated and the wrist is
away from neutral.

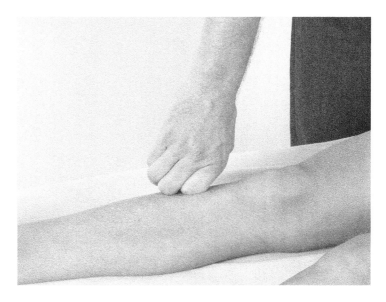

extremely painful, if not fully inoperable. I've known some excellent Shiatsu
therapists who did long-term damage to the thumb in this way (Fig. 5.11).

Figure 5.11
Incorrect: good palpation
tools but not useful for
MFR or any transmission
of force.

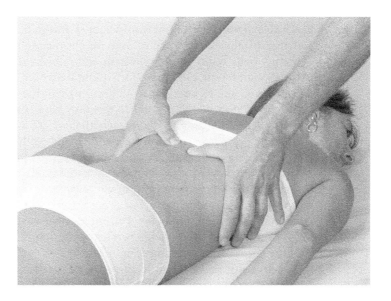

At times, having the thumbs in this hyperextended position can be
useful when palpating. For example, the thumbs work well to assess the
relative position of the transverse processes, other bony landmarks or soft
tissue tone.

For good support, keep the thumb snug against the first finger, which in
turn is held in the 'soft fist' position. This provides a great deal of stability with
no strain to the carpometacarpal joint and surrounding ligaments (Fig. 5.12).

Figure 5.12
Correct: the thumb is protected from any strain at the MC joint.

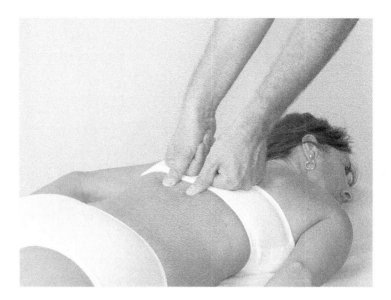

EFFECTIVE FULL BODY USE

Most manual therapists are given at least basic instruction on body mechanics in their courses. While the quality of this input varies a great deal, one recurring theme is the need to use bodyweight rather than muscular effort where possible. This is useful but insufficient. For instance, it fails to address the fact that transmitting the force of bodyweight through the upper extremity into a client's body requires an equivalent amount of work to be done in stabilizing the shoulder joint and girdle. Otherwise we would lean into our work through our hands only to have our shoulders move in the opposite direction and render the contact ineffective. Since this only happens to a small extent, it's clear that we are stabilizing that joint, whether we are aware of it or not.

There are necessary additions to be made to this advice about gravity. Try working with the hip hinge as the primary axis of movement for lowering the bodyweight towards the client. At the same time, maintain an awareness of the sacrum and coccyx dropping down, away from the movement of the head, which is reaching forward. (For more information on the value of reaching in a specific direction, see below.) Bringing your weight forward in this way will contribute to an overall lengthening of the spine, with an associated opening of the chest, while working (Fig. 5.13).

Activating the hip, while allowing the coccyx to 'reach' in the opposite direction to the contact being made with the client, will enable the therapist to elongate the hamstrings, lengthen the front line of the trunk and maintain access to the diaphragm. Working in this manner means the therapist can be exploring internal space, stability and elongation during treatments! The same attitudes can be brought to work done from the seated position (Fig. 5.14).

This has to be better than getting locked into exaggerated thoracic kyphosis, with accompanying internal rotation of the humeral heads, dropped clavicles, depression of the upper ribs, exaggerated cervical flexion with associated capital extension, a posterior pelvis, short hamstrings and disconnection from the feet and ground (Figs 5.15 & 5.16).

Figure 5.13
Correct: the hips are engaged as the major point of flexion while the spine is stable, elongating and dynamic.

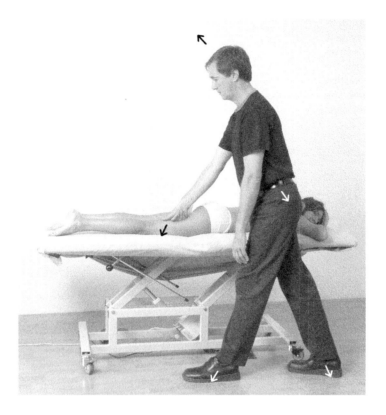

Figure 5.14
Correct: seated position enables the same sense of support, direction and span.

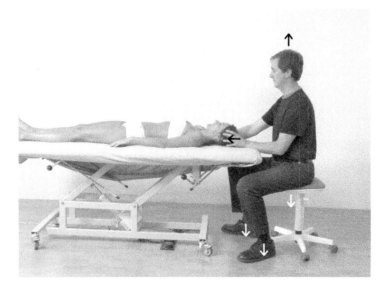

Try to get the pelvic and shoulder girdles facing in the same direction as much as possible. Too much counterrotation between the two girdles can cause facet joint pain and stiffness in the thoracic and lumbar spines, asymmetrical muscle tone and even functional scoliosis – a surprisingly frequent set of problems brought on by the work of manual therapists.

Figure 5.15
Incorrect: loss of support
and direction leads to an
overall shortening of the
therapist's body. Resting
on the elbows forces the
shoulders into the ears.

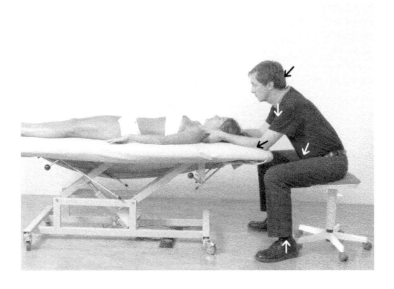

Figure 5.16
Incorrect: loss of support
and direction leads to
shortening and collapse.

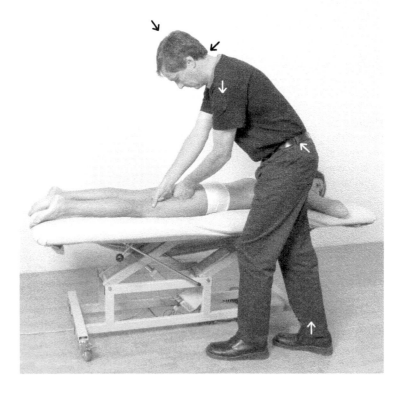

Working from a position of support means much more than saving our bodies from excessive wear and tear. Doing direct technique MFR is about communication. When there is ease and balance in the body of the therapist, this is transmitted to the client as clear intention and a purposeful, responsive touch. This same attitude of economy of effort frees up energy for the therapist to feel, or in other ways sense, the variety of responses of the client to the input they are receiving. This dynamic feedback loop is at the heart of doing good therapy. Establishing a consistency in economical body use goes a long way toward cultivating this potential.

An experiment

Try this simple experiment. Stand beside a friend whose shoulder should be flexed to 90° with the elbow extended. Grasp their arm and attempt to push it toward the ground while asking them to resist (Fig. 5.17). Both persons should note the effort involved.

Figure 5.17
Stability attempted without direction.

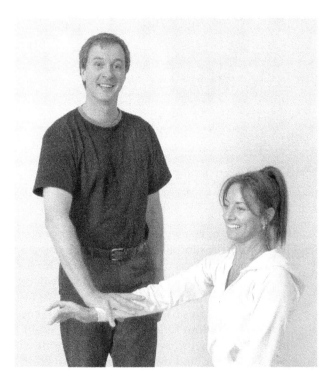

Try again but this time the person with the extended arm 'reaches' with their intention to a point on the wall behind you or even through the wall. In other words, they have a specific sense of direction rather than simply resistance. Generally, the pusher will find the arm much harder to push down while the reacher will feel much stronger and more stable (Fig. 5.18).

What is happening here? And how does this 'Karate Kid' energy stuff help us in our work? Although it's beyond the scope of this book to fully explore the neurology of this cute parlor trick (some of you may have already come across it in schools of chi development and so on), it can be said that movement made with a sense of direction recruits the appropriate muscles but not their antagonists. The first movement, where effort was made to resist the downward force, without any deliberate direction, generates a high degree of contraction in the agonist and the antagonists. The muscles work against each other and effectively weaken in a mistaken attempt to make stronger.

The Feldenkrais teacher Ruthy Alon suggests that these kinds of contractions involve what she terms 'parasitic' muscles whose involvement we are not

Figure 5.18
Stability with a deliberate
sense of direction.

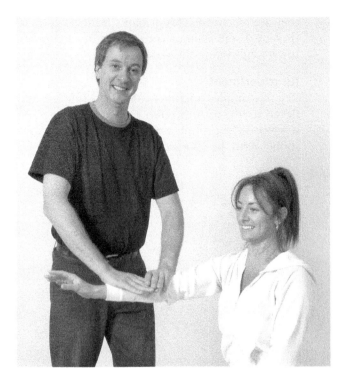

usually aware of as they are habitual and not easily brought into awareness.[1] These automatic subroutines are generally going on all the time and they interfere with many aspects of balanced tonus.[2] This is a shot-gun approach to muscle contractions; getting everything to fire will certainly move something but without finesse. And with fatigue.

For therapists this has far-reaching consequences, if you'll pardon the pun. As we do the various actions to explore the positions suggested above, we can add another dimension that will significantly diminish the effort we make as we work. It's about direction rather than effort. If you work into the myofasciae of the hip triangle but think about reaching through that anatomic region into the table or through to the floor (or the center of the earth?), you add direction. The muscular effort will diminish while the effectiveness of your work will increase. While this can be hard to learn – the Protestant work ethic may have captured vast tracts of your nervous system – it can happen if you pay attention to it. Think direction rather than wrestling match.

The process of decompressing and releasing is a potential in the client's body. The best way to activate it is to communicate with just the right amount of effortlessness. Zero effort and you have, perhaps, energy work, Reiki and the subtlest ends of the cranial spectrum. This might not be the agreement for therapy that you have made with your client. Too much effort and you can be gouging, ripping or thumping. This is probably not the agreement for therapy that you have with your client either. (Please, really, no ripping or thumping, ever.)

If you like this fun game then it can be developed in other ways. While standing, and before making contact with the arms/fingers/elbows onto the client, find, clearly, the awareness of your feet. This is all about sensation – temperature, pressure and texture can each be contacted. Then extend this into an imagined sense of being supported at a point about a meter below you – or the center of the earth if you have a good imagination – rather than at the floor and allow your imagination to take your awareness through to that point. The first time it may take a few seconds; subsequent visits take much less. Note the relative sense of support when contrasting this more deliberate direction-specific connection with your normal habit. One consistent feature of the sensation-rich approach to orienting against gravity is a sharp reduction in tiring patterns of muscular co-contraction.

For the technique driven this can appear to be a frivolous diversion from the real tasks of manual therapy. Of course, some people are blessed with a naturally flexible, robust nervous system. Many are not, though. I see many clinicians who are fatigued from doing soft tissue work with a lot of over-exertion. A friend calls work like this white collar laboring. The burnout rate amongst the manual therapy laboring class is, regrettably, very high. Perhaps there's a place here for the old 'Work smarter, not harder' maxim, given here with some hints that may allow it to integrate into your working days.

So … feeling tired or crunched in a session? Disconnected? Check and see if you've lost sensory awareness of your feet/hands/back/head. Orient to sensation and then add direction to feet/hands/back/head and see if this unwraps you without any big attempt to adopt correct form (remember the wasted effort made in the unbendable arm game).

I suspect that many of the really fine manual therapists who contact their clients across a spectrum of levels, from the energetic to the dense, are engaged with this type of low-effort, direction-specific contact. Milne describes his approach to cranial work in the beautifully titled '*The Heart of Listening*'.[3] This book is rich in the kind of evocative imagery and metaphoric language that can shift us away from the hard yards of soft tissue slug fests in 'resistant tissues'. One can see how this style of sensation-rich contact, married with a sense of direction, could lead us to a new appreciation of what it means to touch, work and listen at the same time. This kind of dynamic, of saying hello through touch and listening for the response, is central to what this book is about.

COMMENTS FOR PEDIATRIC THERAPISTS

In the pediatric settings where I work, we treat children all over the place – floors, wheelchairs, cradled in the mother's arms, mats on conference tables, and so on. Rarely have I worked on anything resembling a true treatment table, adjusted to the correct height for my body. Electric height-adjustable tables seem even less common.

The most common place is a mat on the floor. Take care of your own body when working on the floor. I've found it's easy to start feeling crunched after spending a few hours doing MFR down there. Then the quality of touch starts to change. Contact made with a clear sense of direction on the part of the therapist is often replaced, at best, by the 'application of a correct technique'. The hand holds will be right, the anatomic structures being touched are correct but the communication changes. Mechanical pushing into the intrafascial mechanoreceptors replaces a sustained 'hello'. Enter the Law of Diminishing Returns: the harder you work, the less effect it seems to have.

Learning how to maintain a stable core is important for everyone. For manual therapists and somatic practitioners who spend a lot of time as 'floor workers', it is essential. Working in the standing position makes it easier to engage and work from the core stabilizers. This is because of the closed chain kinetic connection through to the feet. Working on the floor, this chain is then opened, which results in movement with increased amounts of co-contraction. Large phasic muscles are used as stabilizers. This is tiring, exhausting even.

In my highly informal straw polls taken in the various classes I teach, pediatric therapists report a higher incidence of SIJ and lumbar pain than other therapists. I suspect that this is associated with the failure to successfully stabilize the pelvis, sacrum and lumbar spine due to the amount of time spent in the open chain relationship to gravity. It might also have something to do with the fact that the majority of pediatric therapists are women. Many have had children, another contributing factor to weakening of the deep abdominal stabilizers. These suggestions for better body use may be helpful no matter what the underlying cause of the instability may be.

Work in a dynamic two-point kneel. This closes the chain. Augment this by dorsiflexing the back foot sufficiently to get the toes on the floor rather than resting on its dorsal surface in a passive plantarflexed position. Reach/step through to the toes to initiate forward movement into the hands. This activates the same vital connection between the foot and thoracolumbar fascia as walking. This is where the support for the low back can come from.

Test the difference. Pay attention to the hips, the internal spaces of the pelvis and the breath while doing this. Do the movement as described, with the toes on the ground and the plantar surface of the foot on slight stretch. Reach into the back foot while extending both arms into the floor/pillow/person, etc. Now drop the foot into plantarflexion and make the same forward-reaching motion through into the hands. Generally, the first approach will leave the hips feeling loose and open, also the pelvic floor and breath. In the second approach, the hip muscles will have to stabilize the pelvis, leading to feelings of restriction there as well as in the breathing. This can easily be verified by attempting to 'wag your tail' while in each position (Fig. 5.19).

Figure 5.19
Body position for stability while working on the floor.

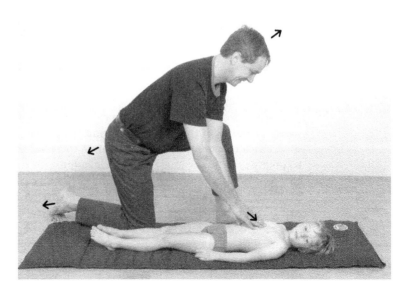

Try working from a kneeling bench – a heavy-duty meditation cushion is used in Figure 5.20. While this is not as dynamic as the two-point position described above, it offers advantages over sitting cross-legged, mainly that the knees are lower than the hips, leaving the pelvis free to find an easy neutral position. Sitting cross-legged, where the knees are invariably higher than the hips, pushes the pelvis into posterior tilt, quite often to an extreme degree. Once there, postural stability is almost impossible to maintain, with the spinal erectors eventually exhausted by their efforts. Burning, painful hot spots develop at various sites along the back and in the suboccipital area. These hot spots give the nervous system plenty of noxious stimulation and diminish the chance of discrete muscular balance of the type required for easy posture (Fig. 5.20).

Figure 5.20
Use of a kneeling stool to support stability while treating on the floor.

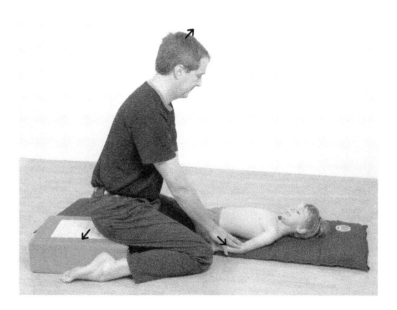

GENERAL POSTURAL STRATEGIES FOR FLOOR WORKERS

- Keep the waistline at neutral as much as possible. Avoid pulling up into hyperlordosis or crunching over into lumbar kyphosis.
- Feel the spine as long without forcing it – the coccyx drops down and the top of the head lifts up. (Waistline at neutral!) This works especially well when there is a closed chain situation in the lower extremity but can certainly be explored at all other times.
- Allow the back of the head to feel wide and the suboccipital triangle to open.
- Soften the gaze frequently. The effect of this is amazing. Really. Try it.
- Stay sensory; notice texture, temperature, pressure, light, shadow, color and shape. 'Coming to our senses' is one of the most central components of changing posture. This is not labored, serious stuff but as simple as noticing in an instant the position of a hand, the feeling of our skin on another's skin, the texture of the carpet, the mortar in the bricks. See Chapter 4 for more on this line of thinking.

References

1. Alon R 1996 Mindful spontaneity. North Atlantic Books, Berkeley, CA
2. Frank K 1995 Tonic function: a gravity response model for Rolfing structural integration and movement integration. Self-published. Available online at: www.somatics.de
3. Milne H 1995 The heart of listening, vols I & II. North Atlantic Books, Berkeley, CA

Section 2
APPLICATION OF TECHNIQUES

Chapter 6
THE LOWER EXTREMITIES

ANKLE RETINACULUM

Client

Sidelying with upper hip flexed to 70° and upper knee flexed to 45°, and supported by a pillow.

Therapist

Standing at the foot of the table.

Technique

Begin directly on the malleolus of the fibula. Use the knuckles, fingertips or thumbs of both hands to sink into the thin layer of tissue over the bone. Take up a line of tension in the fasciae. Carry this line off the bony margins and away from the midline. Spread and melt while the client further engages the release via movement (Fig. 6.1).

Figure 6.1
MFR of the ankle retinaculum showing the spreading of the tissue using two hands.

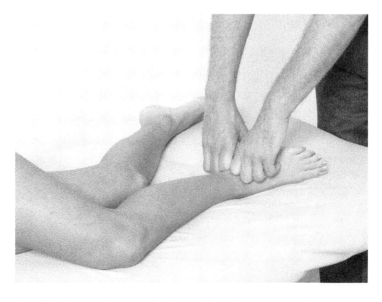

Movement

Dorsiflexion and plantarflexion with a clear sense of direction. 'Bring your toes towards your nose' as an example for dorsiflexion.

Comments

This is a basic release for the lower leg and useful in many situations – fibrous change after trauma, hypertonicity of any of the lower leg muscles or any condition involving decreased ROM at the ankle. Use it also as a prelude to any mobilizations of the talus, fibula or tarsal bones.

ANTERIOR COMPARTMENT/INTEROSSEUS MEMBRANE

Client   Sidelying with upper hip and knee flexed, and supported by a pillow.

Therapist   Standing at the foot of the table.

Technique   Use an elbow with 90° of flexion and begin above the malleolus of the fibula. Glide proximally 2–3 inches at a time between the tibia and fibula. Superficial fascia can be treated more quickly – the interosseus membrane will respond to slow, steady contact. Encourage the client verbally to fully allow the weight of the treated leg into the table (Figs 6.2, 6.3).

Figure 6.2
Using the elbow to release the myofasciae of the anterior compartment.

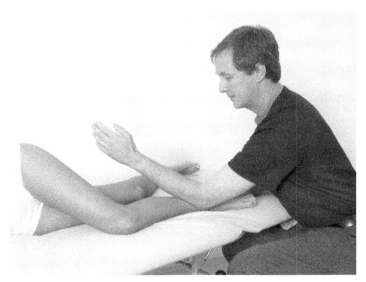

Figure 6.3
Alternative client position and therapist tool (soft fist) for releasing the anterior compartment.

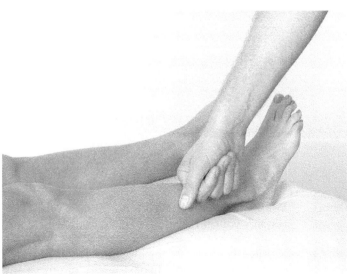

Movement

Dorsiflexion and plantarflexion with a clear sense of direction. 'Lengthen your heel toward the wall/door/painting/vase/skeleton' as another direction-specific example for dorsiflexion.

Comments

Use this in conjunction with the retinaculum release for hypertonicity and fibrous changes in the anterior compartment. Assists with reducing pressure in the compartment. Restores ROM at the ankle. Useful prior to mobilizing the fibula. Chronic stiffness in the lower leg can significantly alter gait and subsequently, SIJ function. Can be combined with the previous release to provide increased sensory awareness to the feet and ankles for gait and balance training.

GASTROCNEMIUS

Client

Prone, with feet off the end of the table to allow for easy dorsiflexion.

Therapist

Work from a stool for technique number 1. Face toward the feet while standing or sitting at the client's side, at around mid-thigh level, for technique number 2.

Technique

1. Use an elbow flexed to 90° and take up a contact in the tendo Achilles. Establish a line of tension in a superior direction. Tether the tissue while the client dorsiflexes. Focus the release at the junction of the tendon and the muscles (Fig. 6.4).

Figure 6.4
MFR of the gastrocnemius using an elbow.

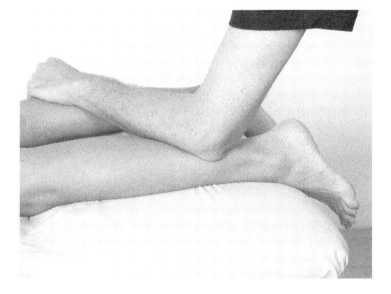

2. Use the index and middle fingers of each hand to take up a contact on the tendons of the gastrocnemius at the epicondyles of the femur. Put a line of tension in an inferior direction and sink slowly into the tendinous structures in the posterior knee. Carry this down into the superior portions of the muscle, which are often highly fibrous. Again, tether the tissue while the client first dorsiflexes (Fig. 6.5).

3. Use the index, middle and ring fingers of each hand to sink into the medial and lateral aspects of the calcaneus. Establish a line of tension in an inferior

Figure 6.5
Finger placement for release of the tendons in the posterior aspect of the knee.

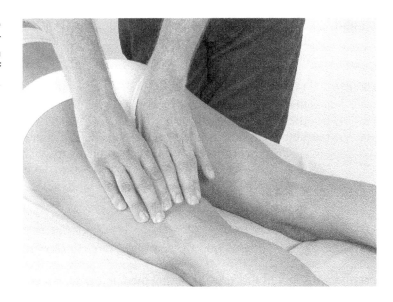

direction and tether the tissue while the client dorsiflexes and then plantarflexes against the resistance (Fig. 6.6). Repeat up to 6–7 times.

Figure 6.6
Finger placement for the release of the fascia at the calcaneus.

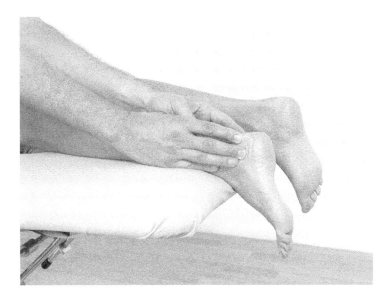

Movement

Dorsiflexion. 'Lengthen your heel away from your tailbone' as an example rather than the more mechanical and directionless 'Flex your ankle'.

Comments

Shortness in this posterior aspect of the lower leg is legendary. Palpate through the muscle bellies and you'll find lengths of vine, string, rope and, occasionally, cable. Release the superficial gastrocnemius before going into the deeper soleus.

SOLEUS

Client

Prone with feet off the end of the table to allow for easy dorsiflexion. Use a bolster to induce 10–15° of knee flexion and put the gastrocnemius off stretch.

Therapist

Sit on a stool at the end of the table, facing towards the head. Standing is also acceptable.

Technique

Use an elbow or fingers to sink into the tendo Achilles. Sink slowly through the tendon into the investing layer of fascia that lies between the soleus and the gastrocnemius. Take up a line of tension in a superior direction and tether the tissue while the client dorsiflexes (Fig. 6.7).

Figure 6.7
Using the fingers to release the myofasciae of the deep posterior leg. Elbow might be better on a large leg.

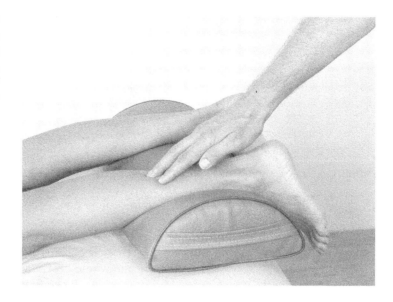

Movement

Dorsiflexion with direction. 'Lengthen the back of your lower leg while paying attention to all of the in-between places in the movement, not just the endpoint' as an example.

Comments

The underlying tissues are made accessible by putting the gastrocnemius off stretch. Go slow on the soleus – it is surprisingly tender in many people. Good release here can transmit all the way through the hamstrings, pelvic floor and into the lower back.

PLANTAR MYOFASCIAE

Client

Prone with feet off the end of the table to allow for easy dorsiflexion.

Therapist

Sitting on a stool at the end of the table.

Technique

Use the knuckles, soft fist or elbow to engage the soft tissue just anterior of the calcaneus (Fig. 6.8). Take up a line of tension in an anterior direction. Work progressively through to the ball of the foot as well as into deeper layers in subsequent passes.

Figure 6.8
Release of the plantar myofasciae using a soft fist.

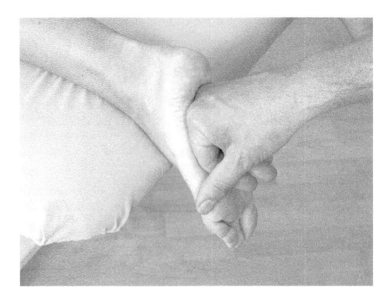

Movement

Have the client lift their toes, with direction – 'Lengthen the bottom of your foot by taking your toes up under the table towards your knee cap'. Dorsiflexion can also be used in conjunction with this.

Comments

This can be done in conjunction with the work into the posterior compartment. Consider using it when there is chronic stiffness and hypertonicity in that region as well as through the whole posterior aspect of the leg and into the back. It will increase proprioception in the foot and ankle which will assist with gait and balance training. Breathing will also be affected by working here. Listen and watch for multiple 'therapeutic breaths'. Often the entire tonus of the person changes as these releasing and integrative breaths occur.

MYOFASCIAE AT ILIAC CREST

Client

Sidelying with lower leg flexed to 30° at the hip and knee. The upper leg is supported on the lower leg but with less flexion at the the hip and knee. The lumbar spine is in neutral.

Therapist

Standing behind the client at the level of their waistline and facing toward the client's feet.

Technique

Use a soft fist to engage the fasciae along the iliac crest. Start at the midline of the coronal plane. Sink inferiorly and then take up a line of tension in a posterior direction (Fig. 6.9). Move across the surface toward the PSIS. Do not attempt

Figure 6.9
Using a soft fist to do
MFR at the iliac crest.

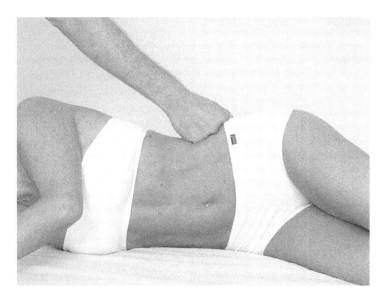

to manually stretch the pelvis away from the rib cage but rather, wait for a tone and texture change that allows the pelvis to drop away without being forced.

Movement

Anterior–posterior tilt of the pelvis with direction. 'Take your tailbone away toward the wall behind you' for an example of anterior tilt. Not surprisingly, given the stiffness in this region, getting this degree of coordination can take some work. Many people have limited or no access to these motions so it is often necessary to stop the manipulation to help educate them about their pelvic motion. Put your hands on the iliac crest and show, by passively moving the bone, the motion you are asking for. Once this is understood, the client can explore this as an active motion.

Comments

Technically, this is of course a release for the pelvis. Still, by crossing major joints, and thus body segments, muscles and fasciae ignore these divisions. I've included it here not as an exercise in postmodern sabotage of agreed-upon anatomic standards but because it works so wonderfully well when done in conjunction with the next two releases. Please revisit it when treating a stiff pelvis!

A number of passes are usually desirable. I call this a 'bread and butter' move in my classes – clients love it for the ease it gives to the breath, low back, SIJ and, often, the whole lateral aspect of the body. Use it before doing deeper work into the quadratus lumborum (QL), the multifidus triangle and any mobilizing of the lumbar vertebrae and SIJs.

On subsequent passes the emphasis can shift to allow for more contact into the area of the QL and the posterior two layers of the thoracolumbar fascia. For this, turn the fist down toward the transverse processes of the lumbar vertebrae.

TENSOR FASCIA LATA

Client

In the same position as for the iliac crest. Make sure they are positioned close to the edge of the table nearest you.

Therapist Standing behind the client at the level of their waistline and facing forward.

Technique Locate the muscle, anterior to the gluteus medius. Use an elbow to sink into it until an obvious barrier to any more depth is encountered. Wait without increasing the pressure. If another layer becomes available, follow it down and wait once again. When there is an obvious and sustained tone change, add a line of tension and move slowly in an inferior direction. The movement across the surface might only be 2–3 cm (Fig. 6.10).

Figure 6.10
Elbow position for treating the tensor fascia lata.

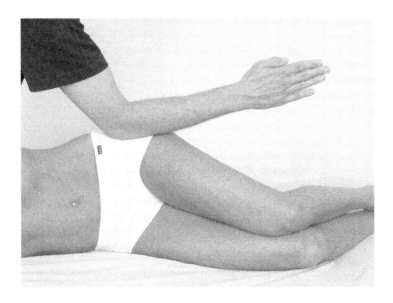

Movement Anterior–posterior tilt of the pelvis with direction. 'Take your tailbone away toward the wall in front of you' as an example of posterior tilt.

Comments Despite sounding like a pleasant frothy coffee drink, this muscle more often feels like cable than liquid.

This release can take several minutes to complete and can be deepened by responding to what you feel under your hands and communicating that to the client. When a tone change occurs then confirm that with them by acknowledging it and suggesting they explore letting go a little more. 'Perhaps there is another layer that you can contact now you can feel the release starting.'

This is an essential work when treating pelvic torsions to assist with restoring balance between the flexors and extensors. It's clearly indicated for helping correct anterior tilts. Congestive conditions of the lower abdominal region – constipation, irritable bowel and painful menstruation – are often helped via this and the following release.

Where needed, the focus can be away from the tensor and more into the gluteus medius fibers. For example, follow a similar protocol of landing and slowly sinking for making entry into the posterior portion of the gluteus medius and then beyond that into the posterior aspect of the greater trochanter to affect the piriformis.

ILIOTIBIAL BAND

Client

As for above.

Therapist

Standing behind the client at the level of their waistline and facing toward the client's feet. Move toward the foot of the table as the release progresses down the leg.

Technique

Use a soft fist or elbow to engage the fasciae at the greater trochanter. As the tissue is relatively thin here, little vertical contact needs to be made before putting a line of tension in an inferior direction. Take this into motion inferiorly along the femur (Fig. 6.11).

Figure 6.11
Using an elbow to release the fasciae at the greater trochanter.

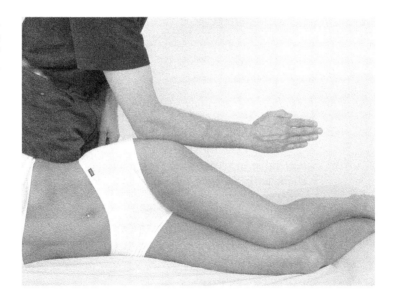

Generally, it works best to divide the band into sections and treat them individually, with a break for the client in between the contacts. Treat all the way to the tibia (be sure to cross below the knee) (Fig. 6.12).

Movement

Anterior–posterior tilt of the pelvis with direction. 'Take your tailbone away toward the wall behind you while gently stepping into your heel' for an example of anterior tilt that helps differentiate the leg from the pelvis.

Comments

This is a notoriously painful area yet my experience shows that the therapist's attitude is the most significant contributor to this. Go slow, work well within tolerance and the tissue will open without any trouble. In fact, the client will usually 'purr' when this release is done properly. A consistent response of guarding, sharp inbreaths, breath holding or even feisty language strongly suggests that the work is too deep.

'Topographic' changes in the ITB are common. Thickening and fibrosity generally increase closer to the knee. It may be useful to come to the front of the table to treat this bottom third of the band. When working here it can be

Figure 6.12
MFR of the ITB using an elbow.

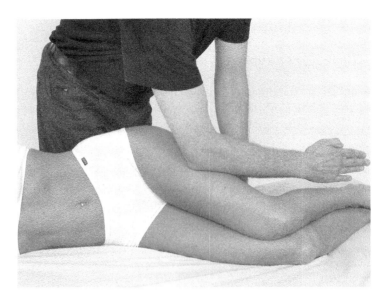

useful to ask the client to fully, and slowly, extend their knee while simultaneously engaging in a mindful pelvic tilt.

Some of the most restricted sites can require multiple treatments. This is preferable to trying to get them all in one session as overtreating can leave the client with a loss of support and a feeling that they are buckling at the knee when standing.

MEDIAL HAMSTRINGS

Client

Prone with feet off the end of the table. If the muscles are very short then bolster the ankles to take the muscles off stretch.

Therapist

Standing on the same side as the muscles being treated, except for the tendons of the medial hamstrings, when working from the opposite side provides a better angle of contact.

Technique

1. Begin at the musculotendinous zone of the 'semis' about 4–5 cm above the knee. Use an elbow, fingers or knuckles to take up a line of tension superiorly and work incrementally towards the ischial tuberosity. Explore the space between the 'semis' and gracilis; treat where needed. At the tuberosity, reduce the angle of contact to around 15° or less. Work up across the tuberosity and into the gluteal fascia as well as the sacrotuberous ligament. If working superiorly is too effortful then bring the contact superior to the tuberosity and sink down into the tendons while maintaining a steady contact against the bone (Fig. 6.13).
2. From the opposite side of the table use the fingers, knuckles or a well-controlled elbow to make contact at the same site as before (4–5 cm above the knee). Sink firmly into the tendons and develop a line of tension towards the feet.

Figure 6.13
MFR of the medial hamstring. Fingers used here for clarity of position in the photo. An elbow would be better.

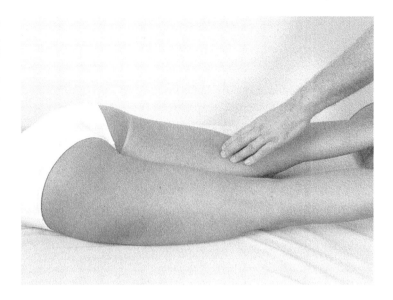

Follow this line across the posterior aspect of the knee. Avoid the popliteal fossa and its associated neurovascular bundle (Fig. 6.14).

Figure 6.14
Using the fingers to release the distal tendons of the medial hamstrings.

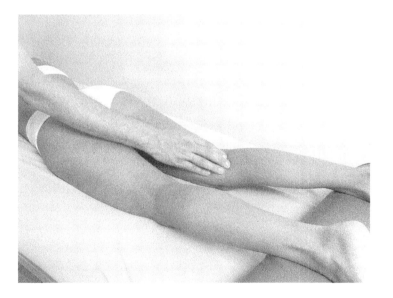

Movement

Anterior tilt of the pelvis with direction. 'Take your tailbone toward the ceiling while you gently lengthen your leg from the heel' for an example of anterior tilt that, once again, helps differentiate the leg from the pelvis.

Comments

Hypertonic and fibrous hamstrings appear to be an epidemic, especially in men. Restoring length and pliancy can ease SIJ and lumbar restrictions as well as improving gait and balance and reducing tibial torsions. Include this work when treating the sacrotuberous ligaments, posterior pelvis tilts, pelvic torsions and sciatic nerve restriction with piriformis involvement as well as restoring normal tone in the pelvic floor.

BICEPS FEMORIS

Client

As for above.

Therapist

Standing on the same side as the leg being treated, at the level of the client's waistline.

Technique

1. The belly and origin of biceps femoris can be treated using the same protocols as for the 'semis' (Fig. 6.15).

Figure 6.15
MFR of the lateral hamstrings using an elbow.

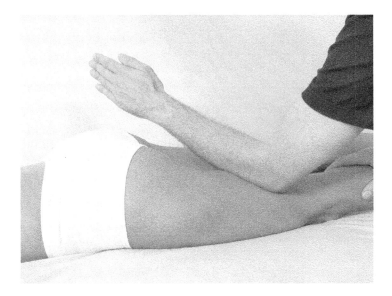

2. The distal tendon can be treated in the same manner as the 'semis'. Follow the line of tension down to the head of the fibula (Fig. 6.16).

Figure 6.16
Using the knuckles to release the distal tendons of the lateral hamstrings.

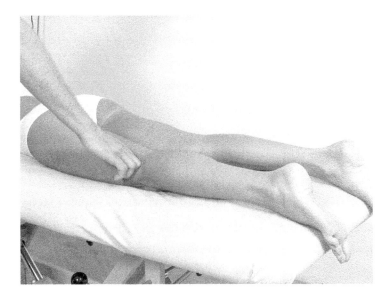

Movement

As for the 'semis'.

Comments

The posterior aspect of the upper leg is a good place to explore palpation skills. Use a flat, soft hand to test for the mobility of layers and the overall tension in the tissue. Do this by placing the hand flat onto the leg. Engage the tissue with around 30 grams of force. Move the tissue in a number of directions, mentally noting when bind is encountered. Using the same flat hand, sink into the tissue with the intention of springing the tissue – a kind of trampoline test. Again, only sufficient force to test for the tensioning and recoil of the tissue is used. This is often much less than we think. Retest with both approaches after treating. The confirmation of change is immediate and, importantly, can be felt by the client as well. This is a chance – there are, of course, many others – to establish that changes in length, pliancy and texture are actually possible through manual therapy. This can be a new concept for many people who have learnt, regrettably, to think of their bodies as unchanging, unfriendly machines that drag them around from place to place.

Extend this style of work into any other areas in the posterior leg that present as stiff and fibrous. This kind of joyful exploration, discovery and subsequent friendly meeting with the local residents of an area is always appropriate. Initially, a treatment might be guided by the descriptions in this book. Curiosity and good palpation skills will find fertile zones for work that do not conform to these guidelines. With the hamstrings, a common line of fascial restriction is between the medial and lateral hamstrings. Another zone to take a look into is between the 'semis' and the adductors. Here you can discover many forms of myofascial congestion, often associated with a great tenderness. Go slow.

Prone position also gives good access to the posterior aspect of adductor magnus. This myofascia is often bunched tight up against the pelvis. Release here feeds superiorly into the pelvic floor and inferiorly into the entire posterior aspect of the leg. Clients often report feelings of space and ease around the sacrum, coccyx and lumbosacral area after this release (Fig. 6.17).

Figure 6.17
Using the fingers to release the posterior aspect of the adductors.

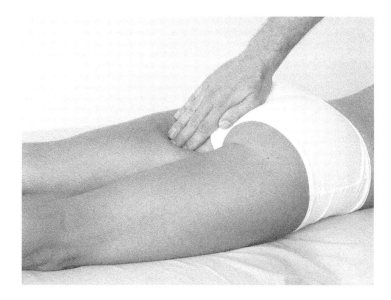

ADDUCTORS

Client

Sidelying with lower leg extended at the hip and flexed at the knee to around 30°. The upper leg is flexed to 45° at the knee and hip. Position client with their back close to the edge of the table nearest you.

Therapist

Standing behind the client, facing headward, at about the level of the feet.

Technique

1. Begin just above the medial epicondyle. Sink into the first layer of restriction, followed by a line of tension in a superior direction. Use an elbow, soft fist or well-supported fingers. Treat in increments, dividing the leg into 3–4 zones of contact (Figs 6.18, 6.19). Initially, work on the midline and then

Figure 6.18
Position of the fingers to release the distal portion of the adductors.

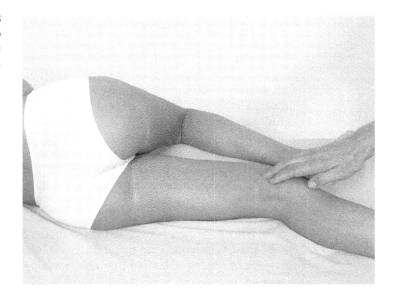

Figure 6.19
Using a fist to release the mid-section of the medial thigh.

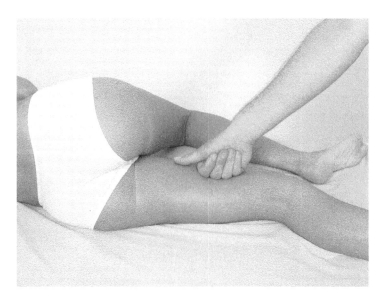

emphasize other areas according to need. Getting close to the pelvis means more myofasciae to work through. Work more deeply as the layers become available. When working slowly, the psoas insertion can be contacted at the lesser trochanter.

2. Use the fingertips to sink slowly into the fasciae along the ramus of the ischium. The initial contact is with the whole hand into the adductor compartment. Then the hand is moved, without gliding across the surface of the leg, in a superior direction until the middle finger contacts the bone. There is only a thin layer and it responds best to sustained contact rather than forceful. Allow the finger to buckle slightly and the index and ring fingers may also make contact (Fig. 6.20). Often, the response takes 45–90 seconds. Maintain the

Figure 6.20
Using the fingerpads to contact the ramus of the ischium.

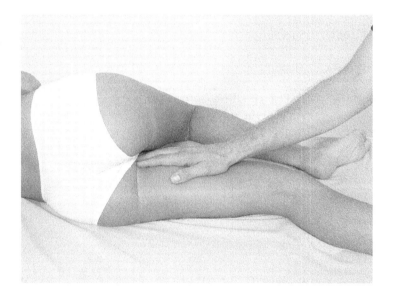

contact for up to 3–4 minutes if the release continues. The response can be felt by the client as an unwinding in the pelvic floor and even as high as the respiratory diaphragm. A common report is an overall sense of relaxation in the viscera.

Movement

When in the adductors, ask for mindful lengthening, 'with direction' movements that involve anterior–posterior tilt.

When working up against the ischial tuberosity, ask for awareness of the breath coming to meet the fingers.

Comments

This is a tender and guarded area on many people, because a number of factors combine to create stiffness and high tone. The proximity to the femoral artery means a primitive protective response; it's on the medial aspect of the leg and covered by deep layers of muscle for a reason, so when we work there we are asking for a shift from reflexive guarding to opening. Psychosexual issues are wrapped around the myofasciae here and may contribute to the tightness.

Clarity of purpose from the therapist needs to be conveyed via some verbal introduction to the technique and what it involves. A confident, non-invasive touch is easily developed if the anatomy is well understood and the beneficial effects of the work have been tracked over a number of clients. The first is easily mastered by reviewing the anatomy in a good atlas. Like all aspects of manual therapy, the second takes time and is basically a numbers game: the more you do, the better you get. I use this work at the floor of the pelvis with many low back and SIJ clients. Signs that it is indicated include inability to isolate the movement of anterior–posterior pelvic tilts in either sitting or lying supine with the related condition of a poor sense of pelvic and lumbar position when sitting and no breath response in the pelvis while lying (prone or supine). The release of a pelvic floor in spasm is a powerful component of restoring normal function to the low back and SIJs.

QUADRICEPS/ANTERIOR ASPECT OF THIGH

Client

Supine.

Therapist

Standing at the client's side at hip level.

Technique

1. Use an elbow or soft fist to engage the tendinous tissues inferior to the ASIS. Take up a line of tension in an inferior direction. Work incrementally toward the knee, dividing the zone into 3–4 segments (Fig. 6.21).

Figure 6.21
MFR of the quadriceps using a soft fist.

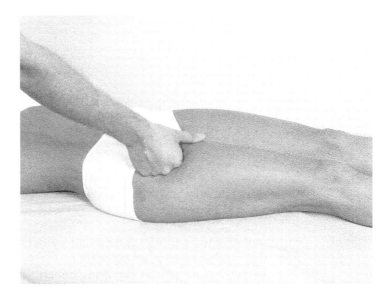

2. Abduct the leg to 15°. Use the fingertips or an elbow to sink slowly into the myofasciae of the femoral triangle. Sink into the tissue in a posterior direction and then take the line of tension in the same direction as sartorius (Fig. 6.22).

Locate the greater trochanter and the ITB. Palpate for the seam between the ITB and vastus lateralis. Take up a line of tension in an inferior direction (Fig. 6.23). Once again, treat incrementally.

Movement

Ask for hip hiking on the ipsilateral side so that the femur moves superiorly, against the line of force moving inferiorly, with direction. 'Lift the hip towards

Figure 6.22
Release of the myofasciae
of the femoral triangle.

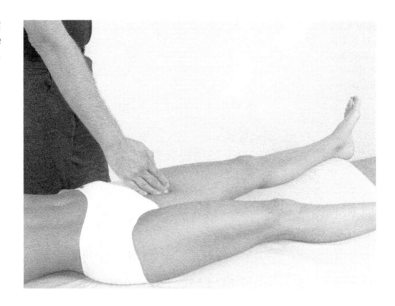

Figure 6.23
MFR of the fascial seam
between the ITB and
vastus lateralis using the
fingers.

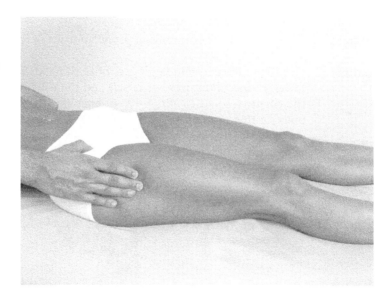

your shoulder while stepping down through the heel on the same side.'
A mindful, 'with direction' posterior tilt is useful to augment work in the
femoral triangle.

Comments   Use all three of these releases in conjunction with the tensor fascia lata release
to assist with correcting an anterior innominate. This can be part of a sequence
to treat pelvic torsions where the anterior tilt is affected via releasing the hip
flexors and the posterior tilt via treating the hamstrings and hip rotators.

The tensor fascia lata is usually tight and fibrous in runners. A Thomas test
will often reveal not only a tight psoas but shortened quads and ITBs as well
(Fig. 6.24). When all three are positive we can safely say that this is not a leg
functioning at its best!

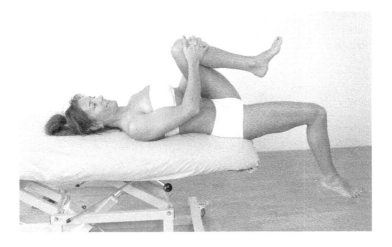

Figure 6.24
The Thomas test. The lumbar spine is flat, not flexed. This photo shows a tight psoas.

STANDING RELEASE: FOREFOOT

Client   Standing with feet hip width apart.

Therapist   Kneeling on the floor, or lying prone, in front of the client.

Technique   Use the index and middle fingers of both hands to take up a contact on the fascia/retinaculum over the tarsals and then the metatarsals (Fig. 6.25). Ask the client to squat to about 45° of knee flexion while you work in counterpoint to that motion with a line of tension that is directed posteriorly. Spread and ease the tissues. The client performs 5–6 squats while the therapist maintains the line of tension.

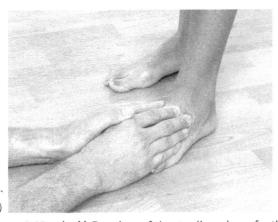
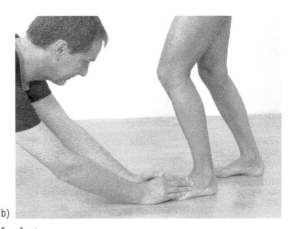

(a)   (b)

Figure 6.25   **(a, b)** Two views of the standing release for the forefoot.

Movement   It is important to have the client emphasize the dorsiflexion aspect of their movement and establish a sense of the weight transmitting through the tarsal bones as they go into the squatting position. 'Bring your knees forward over your second toe and allow the weight to follow.'

Comments

Even though the client's motion is resisted, this is not an attempt to absolutely prevent the response traveling through the soft tissue. As with all releases that use the client's synchronized movements, the contact has to feel cooperative and satisfying.

Introduce this release when there has been trauma to the ankle, knee or hip that has resulted in changes to the gait pattern with all the associated muscle imbalance, proprioceptive distortions and fascial shortening. Quite often, these secondary adaptations are more disabling than the original trauma. Standing work encourages a higher level of integration. It calls for balanced, functional movement in the gravitational field and makes new requests from the proprioceptive system, improves coordination and lengthens shortened fascia.

STANDING RELEASE: CALCANEUS

Client

Standing with feet about hip width apart.

Therapist

Kneeling, or lying prone, behind the client.

Technique

Use the index and middle fingers of both hands to take up a contact on either side of the calcaneus. Ask the client to squat to about 45° of knee flexion while you work in counterpoint to that motion with a line of tension that is directed inferiorly (Fig. 6.26). The client performs 5–6 squats while the therapist maintains the line of tension.

Figure 6.26
MFR to the calcaneus –
standing position.

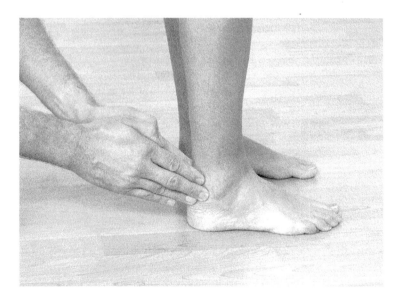

Use the thumb and middle finger of one hand to straddle the forefoot and grasp the anterior aspect of the calcaneus (just below the malleoli). Use the thumb and middle finger of the other hand to grasp either side of the calcaneus on its more posterior aspect (Fig. 6.27). Gently rock the calcaneus from side to side while the client does further knee bends.

Figure 6.27
Hand position for the standing approach to mobilizing the calcaneus.

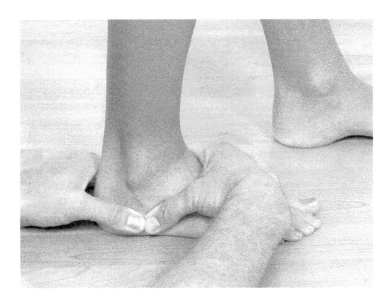

Movement

During all phases of the squatting movement it is important for the client to 'find' their heel and deliberately keep it in contact with the ground. Many people will need instruction on this. Some will lift their heels at the commencement of the motion while others will do so toward end range so as to get further down. In returning to standing, ask them to direct their intent into pushing away through the feet into the ground rather than doing whatever is habitual (and unconscious). This will further awaken the nervous system to new behaviors.

Comments

This can be quite painful if done too aggressively. The therapist's position during the release means that the non-verbal signs of discomfort cannot be observed. Stay in verbal contact instead. Many of the same comments made for the forefoot apply.

STANDING RELEASE: ADDUCTORS

Client

Standing with feet about hip width apart.

Therapist

Kneeling, or sitting on a stool, beside the client.

Technique

Use the fingerpads of both hands to grasp the adductors about a hand's width below the ramus of the ischium. Sink into the tissue by pulling toward yourself. Take up a line of tension in an inferior direction (Fig. 6.28). Ask the client to flex their knees to around 30°. As they return to standing, maintain the intent of the line of tension and work in counterpoint to their movement. Repeat at 2–3 more sites down to the knee.

Movement

During all phases of the squatting movement it is important for the client to 'find' their heels and deliberately keep them in contact with the ground. Many people will need instruction on this. If they are pronated, ask them to emphasize

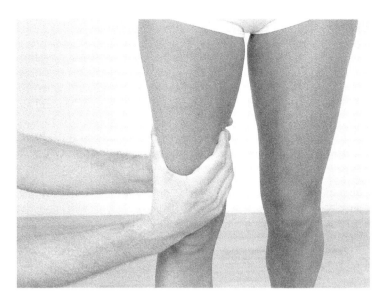

Figure 6.28
Standing approach to releasing the adductors.

the weight on the outside of the foot; for supination, ask for direction of weight to the medial aspect instead. In other words, suggest movement awareness that is non-habitual.

Comments

This looks more like a wrestling match than it is! The line of tension does not have to be deep to be effective. Steady, sustained pressure and a measured resistance to the standing movement are the keys to success.

I've found this to be highly effective for giving lift through the pelvis floor and up into the fasciae of the viscera. It's also useful for derotating the femurs. For internal rotations, where the adductor compartment will be facing more posteriorly, put the line of tension in an anterior–inferior direction and untwist the myofasciae. For an externally rotated femur, where the adductors will be facing anteriorly (a common look on ballet dancers), drag the tissue posterior and inferior.

I use all of the standing work after I have done the opening and decompressing of long-standing restrictions while the client is out of gravity (lying down). This is clearly the best order for most people as the demands on the body when standing, to simultaneously integrate and release, can be overwhelming if this is the initial response in therapy. Some people have a high level of coordination and can move to this standing approach very readily. Others need a lot of work on the table before they can relate to it in a meaningful way.

PEDIATRIC SUPPLEMENT FOR LOWER EXTREMITIES

HAMSTRINGS

Client

Supine.

Therapist

Kneeling, if working on the floor, or standing at the level of the waistline.

Technique

Lift the leg to be treated and allow the knee to passively flex to a non-forced end-range while also taking the hip into flexion. Stabilize the knee with one hand and use the other hand in a soft fist position to sink into the hamstrings just proximal to the knee. The direction of entry will vary according to the degree of restriction in the hamstrings and when the end-range is encountered. Take up a line of tension towards the pelvis and slowly move in that direction. The stabilizing hand is guiding the leg into further hip flexion as the release is generated (Fig. 6.29). In small children both hamstring groups will be treated simultaneously. In larger ones, each group can be isolated in treatment.

Figure 6.29
Showing supine position for MFR to the hamstrings.

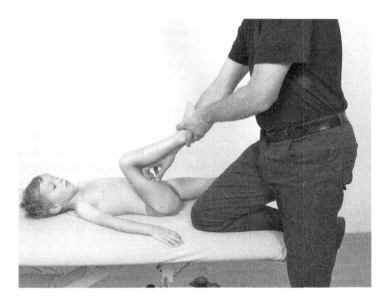

Movement

Generally, in pediatrics, the movements are made passively by the therapist. Sometimes in older children with mild or moderate disabilities, some degree of cooperative motion can be achieved. With this release the hip flexion is increased by the therapist as the hamstrings lengthen.

Comments

This position satisfies my desire to make eye and face contact with the child. Prone position can be unsettling for children because of the absence of this type of contact. There is little effort needed here, just a sustained weight transfer that meets the leg at an oblique angle. Rapid tone changes are common followed by deeper fascial releases. Clearly, this is excellent work for children who are unable to stabilize their pelvises due to high-toned, stiff hip extensors. These releases can augment any neuromotor and developmental approaches to therapy.

POSTERIOR COMPARTMENT – 'HEEL CORD'

Client

Supine.

Therapist

Standing or sitting on a stool at the feet. It is not recommended to do this release on the floor.

Technique

1. Reach with both hands around into the posterior aspect of the leg immediately below the patellar fossa. Support the hands in this position by resting on the elbows and then lift all the fingers in an anterior direction. This will take the contact into the zone of the hamstring/gastrocnemius tendons overlap. The fingers touch each other at the midline. The line of tension is then inferior and spreading to the side in an inverted V shape. The heels of the hands can be used to press the leg into the fingers to increase the engagement. Work incrementally down to the Achilles tendon (Fig. 6.30).

Figure 6.30
Hand and finger placement for MFR to the proximal posterior compartment with the client in supine.

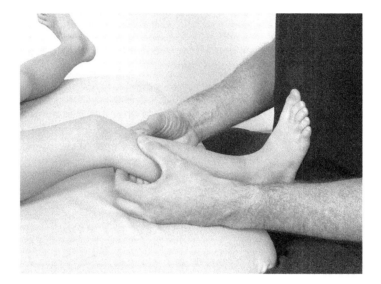

2. Engage the tendon just superior to the calcaneus in the same two-handed manner. The tissue is thin over the bone here so there is a need to pay attention to the quality of the contact – it needs to be as broad and blunt as you can make it, otherwise the child will not be happy. This time the line of tension is inferior without any lateral spreading (Fig. 6.31).

Figure 6.31
Hand and finger position for MFR to the distal posterior compartment. The thumbs are engaging the retinaculum and giving pressure to both sides of the joint.

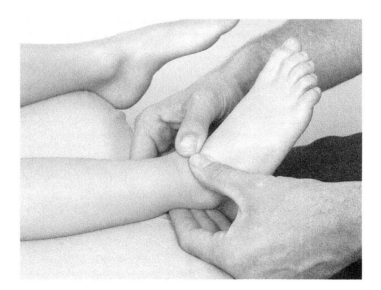

Movement

Working on the table enables the therapist to use their chest or abdomen to lean onto the foot and passively dorsiflex the ankle in counterpoint to the inferiorly directed line of tension. With practice, the therapist can also move the foot into inversion and eversion during this procedure so as to increase the sensory stimulation in the foot and ankle region. The leaning can be quite firm as the sustained sensation of pressure in conjunction with the MFR generally assists in reducing tone.

Comments

Once again, this position satisfies my desire to make eye and face contact with the child. Often, just being supine is sufficient to allay their fear of not being able to monitor the therapist. Or they can be bolstered at the head to make it possible for them to see your face. This work is useful in a range of situations related to gait and balance. It can assist with toe walkers. Scar tissue from tendon releases can be addressed in this position. With scars, you can never go too slowly. Once the line of tension is established then simply wait for the fascia to start its creep. There is often little or no actual movement over the surface. This can also be used in conjunction with the hamstring releases to reduce the tone in the whole posterior aspect of the body.

Chapter 7
THE PELVIS

GLUTEUS MAXIMUS

Client

Prone position.

Therapist

Standing beside the client at the waistline, working on the contralateral side.

Technique

Use the pads of the fingers on both hands to engage the tissues over the PSIS and the intermediate sacral crest. Take up a line of tension toward the greater trochanter (Fig. 7.1). The intention is to contact the fibrous soft tissue over the bones and then take the treatment out into the more muscular fibers of the gluteus muscle. While on the bones the angle of contact is shallow – 15° or so. The angle of contact increases once the more muscular fibers are engaged, perhaps to as much as 45°. Once into the muscle, maintain a consistent depth for each contact that is made. Increase the depth on subsequent passes, as the tissue becomes available.

Figure 7.1
MFR of the gluteal and lower thoracolumbar fasciae and gluteus maximus.

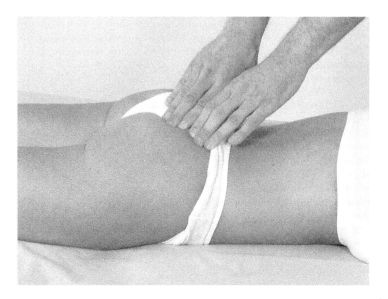

Movement

The client can be encouraged to breathe toward the point of contact. Slight nutation and counternutation of the sacrum – 2–3° – will deepen the effect of the release.

Comments

This release is an important prelude to the deeper work into the sacrotuberous ligament. Many therapists concerned with imbalances between the strength of the gluteus maximus (weak) and the hip flexors (short and tight) see no need for anything but strengthening of this muscle. However, it has been my consistent observation that chronic fibrous changes here are common, even when the muscle would be considered long and weak. These changes are detrimental to the normal function of the muscle and, in my opinion, need to be released prior to any strengthening program. In particular, the tissues lying over the top of the bones need to be released and mobilized as part of any treatment of either the muscle or the SIJs.

Tension is often felt here as tight, cinched buttocks that cannot be relaxed through deliberate inhibition alone. Effective MFR is needed to release these tensions at a reflex level. Quite deep and extremely obvious changes in the tone of the muscle will be observed during the treatment.

SACROTUBEROUS LIGAMENT (STL)

Client

The first technique is done with the client in prone position. For the second position, the client is sidelying, with both legs flexed to 45° at both the hip and knee.

Therapist

Standing behind the client at the waistline.

Technique

1. Work either through the undergarment or directly on the skin. Use an elbow, fingers or a well-supported thumb to sink anteriorly through the gluteus maximus. This is done at a point approximately midway along its attachment to the sacrum and 2 cm lateral. The superficial tissue is often fibrous in this zone and usually deserves full treatment of its own (see previous release). Settle more deeply as the tissue allows for it. Locate the ligament and put a line of tension in an inferior lateral direction, toward the ischial tuberosity (Fig. 7.2).

Figure 7.2
Releasing the sacrotuberous ligament.

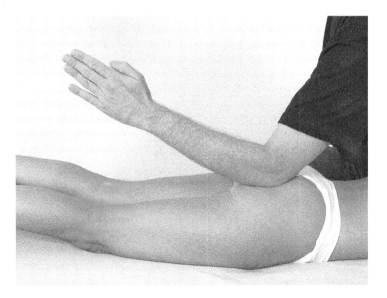

2. Work through the undergarment. Use the pads of the fingers in the area approximately 2 cm lateral and inferior to the coccyx (Fig. 7.3). Sink laterally

Figure 7.3
Using the fingerpads to release the sacrotuberous ligament through the undergarment. Useful when pressure in prone position cannot be tolerated.

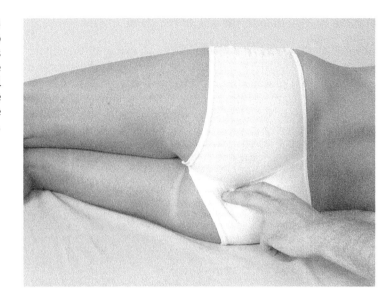

(toward the table). Maintain firm contact in that direction and wait for a distinct sense of softening. This may take up to 2 minutes.

Movement

With the first position the client can internally rotate the ipsilateral leg to give length to the fibers of gluteus maximus. While contacting the STL, lift their lower leg off the table to 90° of knee flexion. Support the leg and guide it into internal rotation. Ask for assistance from the client, with direction – 'Imagine that you are able to roll your foot toward the floor'.

The second position doesn't offer much scope for movement, with or without direction. Asking for mindful attention to the breath is helpful.

Comments

The STL is involved in the normal function of the sacroiliac joints through maintaining an appropriate relationship between the innominates and the sacrum. However, the STL is embedded in the gluteal fascia as well as being an extension of the biceps tendon. Over 30% of the fibers of the biceps cross into the STL without terminating at the ischial tuberosities.

This convergence zone of connective tissues (ligament, fascia, tendon and bone) with contractile tissue (muscle) is often excessively fibrous and stiff. In other words, this is a ligament that has an intimate relationship with many contractile fibers. Like all soft tissue restrictions, there can be numerous and interrelated reasons for these changes – trauma, postural strain, dietary factors and so on. These fibrous changes can contribute (the range of factors is of course larger than this) to a reduction or complete loss of motion at the sacroiliac joint.

The normal amount of movement at the sacroiliac joint is still very much debated. The diagnostic accuracy of many of the standard motion tests – standing stork (or Gillett) in particular – is also under question. While these debates develop a fuller understanding of the joint, soft tissue approaches to easing general myofascial stiffness in the pelvis will continue to improve function and diminish pain.

PIRIFORMIS

Client

Prone position.

Therapist   Standing to the side of the client at waist level.

Technique   **1.** Locate the piriformis by drawing an imaginary line between the midpoint of the lateral aspect of the sacrum and the greater trochanter. Make contact into the gluteus about 3 cm from the sacrum. Use an elbow or a well-supported thumb to sink anteriorly. Engage and wait at the first layer of resistance. Proceed when that layer softens until the fibers of piriformis are contacted. Take up a line of tension along the muscle, in the direction of the greater trochanter. Open the tissue out along this line of tension. Monitor for muscle guarding and moderate the depth of contact accordingly (Fig. 7.4).

Figure 7.4
MFR of the piriformis using an elbow.

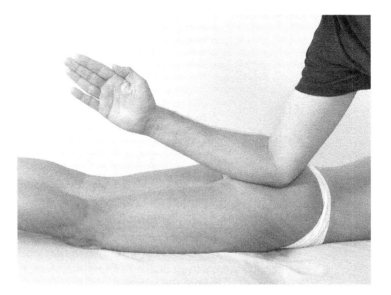

2. While maintaining contact with the piriformis, lift the lower leg off the table to 90° of knee flexion. Support the leg and guide it into internal rotation (Fig. 7.5).

Figure 7.5
Using the client's leg to assist with opening the myofascia of the posterior hip.

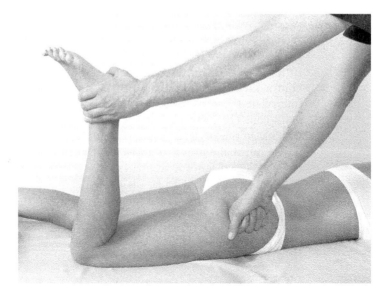

| **Movement** | Ask for assistance from the client with part 2, with direction – 'Imagine that you are able to roll your foot toward the floor'. |

| **Comments** | Piriformis and the sciatic nerve have a close relationship. Using a broad blunt tool like the elbow will be great for releasing the spasmed and/or fibrous piriformis. However, this can irritate the sciatic nerve. I've mostly seen this when the focus is too much on 'stretching' the tissues rather than allowing for the melting and softening effects associated with a slow approach. As always, mindful palpation will enable the therapist to be both effective and safe here. |

OBTURATOR INTERNUS

| **Client** | Sidelying position with the upper leg flexed to 70–90° at the hip and knee. |

| **Therapist** | Standing behind the client at mid-thigh level. |

| **Technique** | Locate the inferior ramus of the ischium on the side of the lower leg. This is approached in the manner used for treating the adductor tendons in Chapter 2 (p65). Spread the contact through the fingerpads rather than simply the tips. Lift the fingers so that the pads move from the inferior surface of the ramus onto its medial (internal) surface. The fingertips will then be extending into the obturator membrane and muscle (Fig. 7.6). A slight amount of further movement (0.5–1 cm) can then be developed. As there is very little scope for creating a line of tension in this small space, the approach is to sink and then wait for a release. |

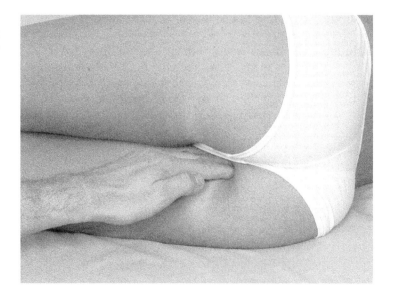

Figure 7.6
Precise finger placement for MFR of the obturator membrane and muscle.

| **Movement** | While maintaining contact with the obturator, ask the client to internally rotate the leg being treated, with direction – 'Roll your entire leg backwards while lengthening through it into your heel'. |

| **Comments** | This release will influence a range of associated structures. Ease can be created in the pelvic floor. The pelvic floor myofasciae are either primary or secondary components of SIJ pain and dysfunction. Prior to teaching core stabilization it is |

necessary to normalize the tissue tone via this release. I have found that all cases of cervical whiplash and many recurrent tension headaches involve spasm of the pelvic floor. Finding ways to effectively release it is essential to resolving these conditions. Changes in the urogenital viscera are common. I recommend this release after bladder infections, for incontinence and painful menstruation. Decompression of the obturator nerve is also possible.

Due to the direct contact into the pelvis, many clinicians will want to have a third person present during the application of this procedure. Those who do not have that option will need to determine what their legal requirements are regarding intrapelvic contact. If it is legal, then a good explanation regarding the logic behind doing the release should be given to the client, supported by an anatomy atlas if necessary. The clinician will also want to gauge the suitability of the release in each specific circumstance that it might be used. For example, if you suspect a borderline personality disorder or other clinical psychological difficulties that involve poor boundaries, then I recommend not using it.

While I greatly favor these direct methods over the classic indirect methods for releasing the pelvic floor, those approaches are useful when the direct method cannot be used.

ILIACUS

Client

Supine with the knees supported on bolsters, if needed, to make the back comfortable.

Therapist

Standing beside the client at hip level.

Technique

Treat one side at a time. Use the fingertips to locate the medial aspect of the ilium at the ASIS. Keep the fingerpads touching the bone (with a slight lateral direction) while the tips sink in an inferior posterior direction (Fig. 7.7). Engage the first layer of restriction and wait. Once release occurs, sink to the next restricted layer and so on. This may take several minutes.

Figure 7.7
MFR for the iliacus.

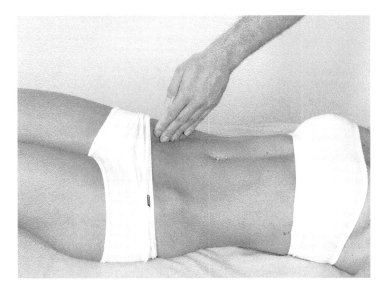

Movement

The client can bring their legs up so that the knees and hips are flexed sufficiently for the plantar surfaces of the feet to be securely on the table. Have them initiate a pushing motion through into the feet that facilitates a slight posterior tilt to the pelvis. The abdomen will drop posteriorly (toward the table) when this is done correctly. Engaging the rectus abdominis to do the tilt will make the abdomen bulge forward. Educate the client about the difference and give a specific direction for the feet to move – 'Push through the table with your feet so that you feel a response in the low back'.

Comments

This release is useful when treating anterior pelvic tilt, either bilaterally or unilaterally if there is a torsion. Other associated structures might also release, particularly tensions in the colon.

PSOAS

Client

Supine with the knees supported on bolsters, if needed, to make the anterior abdominal wall relax.

Therapist

Standing beside the client at hip level.

Technique

Treat one side at a time. Locate the psoas by drawing an imaginary line between the umbilicus and the ASIS. Use the fingers to make contact on this line about halfway between the ASIS and the edge of rectus abdominis. Sink in a medial posterior line (approximately 30° to the surface). Angling in from the lateral edge of the psoas rather than directly over the top of it will avoid jamming the ureters (Fig. 7.8). Once again, engage the first layer of restriction and wait. Once release occurs, sink to the next restricted layer and so on. Eventually the deepest layers will become available but this will take several minutes.

Figure 7.8
Psoas release using direct technique MFR.

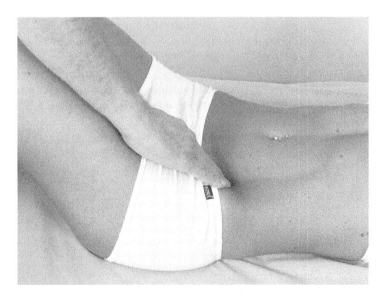

Movement

Let's face it, this release is a 'big ask' for many people. The first time this is performed the focus is generally on tracking the client's responses and working accordingly. Slow. Mindful. Reassuring.

Once the client is familiar with the approach, muscle guarding will diminish and then disappear. It's then possible to involve them in movement.

Have the client bring both knees up. The feet are flat on the table. Tether the psoas in a superior direction while the client slides this leg down onto the table. Attention is given to sliding the foot across the sheet rather than lifting the leg in the air to extend the hip. Pushing through into the foot on the other leg will stabilize the pelvis. Give these instructions with a specific direction and the client will be happily recruiting the appropriate amount of tone to stabilize and move without a lot of parasitic muscle involvement.

Comments

In my classes many people who have already been exposed to a more aggressive approach to the psoas are surprised that working with it is not painful. In fact, done in the way described here, it is most often deeply relaxing and calming. I find that in a high percentage of cases the psoas can be contacted this way. However, some people are unable to tolerate contact at the deep level of the psoas. Significant, counterproductive muscle guarding occurs and does not abate even with time. In these cases I recommend that the region be desensitized over a number of treatments. If ignored, this guarding can develop into an unpleasant autonomic nervous system response and create a strong noxious sensation with nausea as one of the most common effects.

Where desensitization is required, contact whatever level is available – it may be only a few millimeters into the abdomen at first – and allow plenty of time for the client to explore the sensation. Once that contact has been met and understood then another layer may become available. I find it best to develop this increase in depth across three or four sessions. Have other related foci in each session and return here for just a small portion of the session.

This release is indicated when there is increased lumbar lordosis, low back and/or SIJ pain. Done slowly, as detailed here, the work will also assist with the discharge of abdominal stress. Although the reflexive processes by which this occurs are not clear, the activation of the parasympathetic nervous system is consistently observed. Signs include increased borborygmus, slowing of the cardiac pulse, increased salivation and body-wide reductions in tone.

Current trends in lumbar stabilization now include the deepest fibers of psoas as part of the stabilizing core (as well as transversus abdominis, multifidus, pelvic floor, diaphragm). For muscles to function correctly, they must be freed from chronic fascial constriction. I continue to encourage therapists who deal primarily with rehabilitation, and stabilization in general, to include this perspective toward myofascial mobility prior to tone changes when formulating exercise programs.

RECTUS ABDOMINIS (PELVIC PORTION)

Client

Supine with the legs extended. The knees are bolstered to 15° of flexion if the extended position is painful for any reason.

Therapist

Standing at the side at mid-thigh level.

Technique

Treat both sides of the rectus simultaneously.

1. Use the fingertips to engage the lateral margins of the rectus about 2 cm above the pubic bones. Make a 'scooping' motion that begins by first sinking posteriorly into the abdominal wall to engage the aponeuroses of the external oblique (superficial) and the internal oblique (deeper). Once the connection is established, lift under the margins of the rectus to put a line of tension in a medial, anterior and superior direction. This completes the scooping action (Fig. 7.9). Maintain this triplanar line of tension and move superiorly. The client will feel a local stretching sensation at the lower rectus followed by a deeper fascial easing that frees the breath.

Figure 7.9
Working bilaterally on the lower fibers of the rectus sheath.

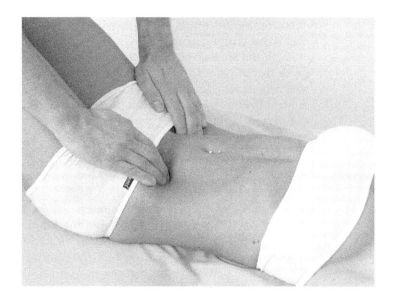

2. Span each iliac crest with the fingers and rest the thumbs on the pubic tubercles. Palpate the pubic symphysis to ascertain tenderness and symmetry between the innominates. The position for palpation is the same as for treatment. Maintain this contact at the anterior superior surface of the pubic bones and spread the contact through the whole of both hands, not just the thumbs (Fig. 7.10). This will direct a good deal of the force – around

Figure 7.10
Using the thumbs to release the rectus abdominis attachments at the pubic bones.

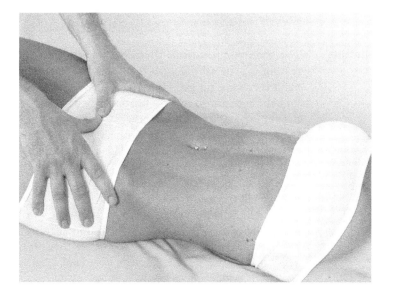

half a kilogram – onto the innominate bones. The direction is posterior. Monitor for changes in fascial tension and muscle tone. The response is usually three-dimensional and feels like the pelvis is opening from the inside out. Re-test for both tenderness and symmetry. Curiously, despite the absence of significant corrective force, there will be a positive change in both measures.

Movement

In the first release, the feet can be brought up to standing position. Ask for slight pelvic tilt with light effort. The emphasis is on allowing the abdomen to relax during this action. The movement is initiated via pushing away into the feet rather than hoisting the pelvis via the abdominal muscles.

With the second release the therapist can shift the palpatory focus by imagining that the hands are hovering half a meter above the body even while the literal contact described above is maintained. This will make the quality of touch quite different. Here we are not 'sinking through' but 'floating above' and for the client it will feel like a broad, unobtrusive three-dimensional sensation that is easily relaxed into.

Comments

Considerable tensions can exist in the myofasciae of the abdominal wall. There is often a strong visual confirmation of this tension with the entire anterior aspect of the trunk pulled short. Release of these tensions is important for asthmatics. Observe the rib cage and respiration during the releases – there will frequently be a significant increase in the excursion of the ribs in unforced inhalation. This can feel deliciously liberating after years of restriction.

The same pattern of fixed trunk flexion can be addressed when treating chronic thoracic stiffness.

PELVIC ROLL WITH LUMBOSACRAL TRACTION

Client

Supine with the knees flexed and the feet flat on the table.

Therapist

Standing beside the client at mid-thigh level and facing toward their contralateral shoulder.

Technique

The therapist positions themselves with one arm between the client's legs, resting on the elbow with the forearm supinated so that the dorsum of the hand is resting on the table (palm up). The client is instructed to push away into the feet and initiate a posterior pelvic tilt. As the pelvis rolls posteriorly, the therapist's arm slides superiorly so that the hand reaches up under the sacrum. The pelvic roll continues so that the lumbar spine starts to go into flexion, one vertebra at a time. This is continued so that the hand can be positioned with the fingertips in the region of L1–L2 (Fig. 7.11). The little and ring fingers will be on one side of the spinous processes, while the middle and index fingers will be on the other.

The client is then instructed to allow the lumbar spine and pelvis to rest back fully onto the hand. By deliberately leaning onto the elbow, the fingers can be made to flex sufficiently to engage the soft tissues in the lamina grooves. This 'lifting' through the fingertips is maintained as the arm is pulled inferiorly,

Figure 7.11
Finger position for engaging the soft tissue of the lumbar spine during the pelvic roll and traction.

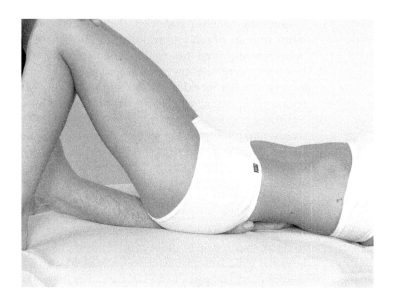

generating a sustained traction through the lumbar region and then the sacrum. Carry the traction out to the coccyx (Fig. 7.12).

Figure 7.12
Client repositioned to show the finger placement for lumbar and pelvic traction.

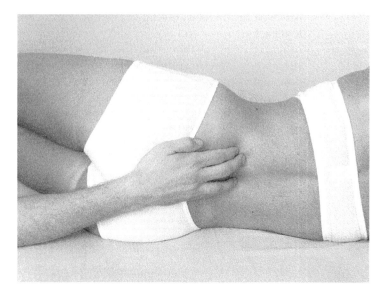

Movement

It is essential to the success of this release that the pelvis rolls rather than being lifted toward the ceiling, often done in an attempt to make room for the therapist's hand. The rolling movement is initiated via a deliberate connection through to the feet, with direction – 'Step down into the whole foot (both) while allowing the abdomen to drop back toward the spine'. Then the hamstrings will naturally activate the motion. The rectus abdominis should not be used. If it is, the effect will be obvious as an unwanted shortening in the front of the waistline. If the rectus abdominis is seen to activate then the therapist's 'free' hand can be placed firmly on the lower abdomen to encourage its relaxation, along with verbal coaching to achieve the desired effect.

Once the hand is positioned, the client is verbally coached to find the maximum amount of relaxation possible. Then the weight of the lower trunk and pelvis is transmitted directly into the therapist's hand. This can take some time but the strong sensory stimulation provided via the fingers and hand will increase the likelihood that the client will naturally send their awareness to that region. This in turn will lead to relaxation and release.

During traction, the client can be verbally coached to continuously allow the weight into the hand. Also verbally encourage release of the posterior pelvic floor ('Relax your bum/buttocks/butt/arse/toosh/hips/keister' – whatever is culturally appropriate!) along with a sense of spreading or releasing across the anterior surface of the sacrum.

Further movement might involve the head which can be guided into an easy rotation and backward bending (spiral motion) with the eyes open and taking in the visual panorama of the room: 'Without any effort, allow your eyes to drink in the shapes, colors and shadows of the corner you are moving your head toward'. This gives a surprisingly rapid spatial reorientation that can be felt as an immediate tone change in the pelvis floor muscles (really!).

Comments

People with low back pain have poor positional awareness. This diminished proprioceptive acuity can be addressed through this release. In fact, while there are clearly biomechanical effects from this traction procedure, the main effect may well be the reawakening of positional awareness – 'Ah, so that's where my low back is! I lost you 5 years ago'. This in turn makes core stabilization and other forms of rehabilitation that focus on coordinated firing patterns more successful. Understanding where we are in space activates the movement potential – 'posture' dictates movement.

Clients will often worry that they are crushing your hand during this release. Reassurance that they are not, that you have done this many times before with persons much larger than they, is important. You might also find that at times your hand *is* being crushed and you're not able to provide any traction at all. If this is truly the case, then focus on the coordinated movement aspect of the release – rolling pelvis, relaxed hips, dropping abdomen, clear sense of segmental motion – and leave your hand out of it.

PEDIATRIC SUPPLEMENT FOR THE PELVIS

ILIAC CREST

Client

Sidelying with the legs at 35° of hip and knee flexion.

Therapist

Kneeling, if working on the floor, or standing – at the level of the shoulders in both instances, in front of the client.

Technique

Use a blunt elbow, making contact on the ulna, distal to the olecranon process. Sink into what will generally be the very thin layer of tissue over the crest at the midline of the coronal plane. Contact this tissue directly atop the superior surface of the ilium. Direct the force in an inferior direction with the deliberate intention of engaging the periosteum as well as the covering tissues.

With this version of releasing the iliac crest there is no line of tension developed. The inferior pressure is simply maintained until the pelvis drops away from the rib cage as part of the change in tone that this release will encourage (Fig. 7.13).

Figure 7.13
MFR to the iliac crest, suitable for the pediatric population.

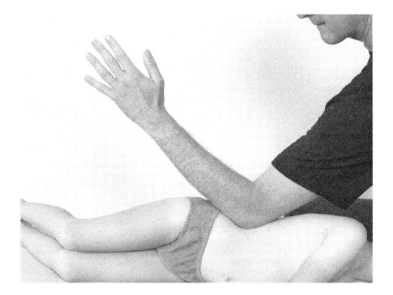

Movement

Nothing specific for this release.

Comments

While this release is covered in the section on the lower extremities (p56), it deserves special consideration in the pediatric pelvis because 'hip hiking' is so common in the cerebral palsy (CP) population. This technique, in conjunction with other releases (hamstrings, hip flexors and adductors), will make a child (or CP or post-CVA adult for that matter) much more available for neuromotor and sensory integration approaches to pelvic stability and positional awareness.

The goal is to be visible to the child while working on them. Although this is not absolutely essential, I favor this relationship with the child whenever possible. However, doing this release from behind the child is also acceptable. Certainly, once deep release has occurred and the child is clearly in a more relaxed and trusting state, then positions other than 'therapist's face visible' can be utilized more readily.

TENSOR FASCIA LATA

Client

Sidelying.

Therapist

Kneeling, if working on the floor, or standing – at the level of the waistline in both instances, in front of the client.

Technique   Use the fingers, a soft fist or an elbow. The pressure should be sufficient to steadily maintain depth without over-exertion. Wait for softening – tone change – and then go more deeply into the tissue. Again, maintain a consistent degree of pressure at that level. If the tone shifts again, follow the opening it makes into the tissue and repeat.

Once the tone has noticeably dropped, a distal line of tension can be introduced that will further lengthen the tissue. This line of tension can be carried anterior to the greater trochanter (Fig. 7.14).

Figure 7.14
Fingers used for MFR to the tensor fascia lata, suitable for the pediatric population.

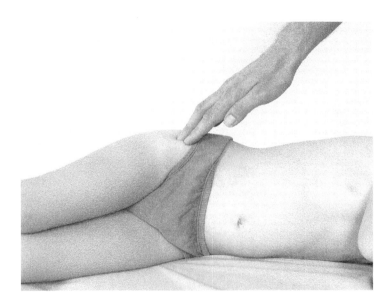

Movement   Once flexor tone is reduced, the other hand can be used to passively take the pelvis through a range of anterior–posterior motion.

Comments   This release is also covered in the section on the lower extremities (p58). It also deserves special consideration in the pediatric pelvis because tight hip flexors are extremely common in the cerebral palsy population.

Once again, the goal is to be visible to the child while working on them.

PSOAS

Client   Supine.

Therapist   Kneeling on the floor at the level of the child's knees and facing toward their head. Or standing at the same level and facing toward the head.

Technique   Hold the leg to be treated in the air to about 30° of hip flexion. Use the index and middle fingers of the other hand to sink into the anterior abdominal wall 1 cm lateral to the ASIS. Angle the contact toward the lumbar spine (Fig. 7.15).

Figure 7.15
Utilizing MFR to the psoas with mobilization of the hip and deep prevertebral fasciae.

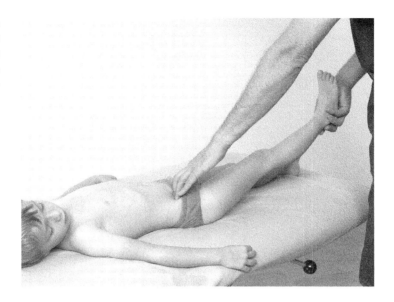

Once the psoas is engaged the pressure should be appropriate to maintain a consistent depth – nothing more.

Initially, the raised (treated) leg is held in a static position. Once some releasing response is detected in the psoas, the leg can be put through a range of motions. These can be internal–external rotation and increased extension as well as abduction–adduction or a combination of all of the above. These are done slowly and the response in the psoas is monitored throughout. The movements should augment the release. A contracted, guarded response would be a sign to reduce the velocity and/or amplitude of the movement.

Comments

Many CP children have hypertonicity in the abdominal muscles as well as the deeper hip flexors. In those instances, the focus should be on releasing these superficial and mid-layer muscles before contact is attempted with the deeper psoas. The lower abdominal release described earlier in this chapter can be easily adapted for a child. Also utilize the upper abdominal release shown in Chapter 8.

With any release in the pediatric population, the position of the child is open to modification. Clearly, where there is a high degree of gamma gain with hypersensitivity of the stretch receptors, attention should be given to finding positions that at the very least do not generate further hypertonicity. For example, it may be necessary to bolster the legs to 90° of hip and knee flexion to make the underlying tissues accessible.

I speak from first-hand experience when I say that any time a treatment starts to develop the feel of a wrestling match, the Law of Diminishing Returns will set in. Yet what defines a wrestling match is also open to modification and reinterpretation based on the situation. For example, I have also found that firm, controlled leaning with parts of the body other than those at the site of the active MFR assists with a general lowering of tone in the high-tone child. This is not a wrestling match. When wrestling develops it is usually at the site of the MFR. It involves a 'you push, I'll push back harder' scenario. With leaning,

Figure 7.16
Making contact with many parts of the body during MFR to the tensor. A leg is resting firmly against the child's back.

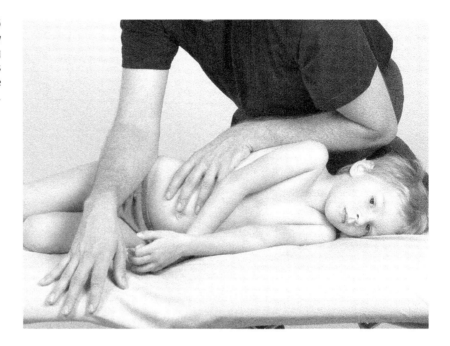

there is a deliberate attempt to deliver a firm, friendly background pressure as well as the local MFR (Fig. 7.16). It can serve to pacify a hyperarousal state as well as take attention away from a more specific contact that may border on noxious if allowed to stand out on its own.

Chapter 8
THE TRUNK

The term 'trunk' has been used here because I find it better than any other existing system of division. The back is often referred to in terms of the lumbar and thoracic spines. These terms are really only about vertebrae. However, they do nothing to help us decide to which zone a muscle or fascia might belong. We might use the dividing diaphragm and the division between the thoracic and abdominal cavities, with structures assigned to one or the other. This might be useful for orienting in visceral work. And both still leave the bulk of the myofasciae without any sense of belonging to one place or another. Which, when we think about it, they don't, as the majority clearly belong to many places at once. So how do I orient to that zone of the body between the neck and the pelvis in such a way that I can talk to you about the soft tissue structures in a coherent, ordered way from my desk in Melbourne, Australia?

I encountered the term 'trunk' being used in pediatric therapy and I liked it. For me, it is an inclusive term and conveys the sense of all that exists between the pelvis and the neck. It suggests three dimensions and brings forth images of trees, with roots and branches to complete the sense of something 'in between'. So while it's not a highly sophisticated term it has its appeal.

To make this next section an applied approach to anatomy, the trunk has been subdivided into the aspects of a person that we work on – back, front and sides. It's simple, I know, but in the end these are what we work on. One could argue that if we include a three-dimensional perspective then there must also be a middle. In this workbook this will be assigned to the section 'deep front'. Of course, the body also has a top (galea aponeurotica) and a bottom (plantar fascia). For now, though, I want to explore the four aspects of the trunk.

In this first section the emphasis is on both the big muscles that cross the entire back, or large sections of it, as well as the smaller ones that are associated more directly with small groups or pairs of vertebrae.

Many of the releases include considerable emphasis on coordination of the whole body in gravity; they are done with the client sitting or, in some instances, standing. These highly coordinated releases are delightful to give and receive – a dance of directions and pressure met, joined and returned. There are also approaches to easing strain in the smaller, intrinsic muscles of the spine. These also require a high degree of coordination and with them the dance is delicate, precise and without any force at all. All in all, it's a big section.

THE TRUNK – BACK

UPPER/MID TRAPEZIUS AND LEVATOR SCAPULA

Client

Seated with attention to the hips being higher than the knees, feet slightly forward of the knees and well connected to the ground. The client is informed that they will support their back via their feet and legs rather than by leaning against the chair's back (if there is one).

Therapist

Either standing behind the client or kneeling on the end of the treatment table. Which option to choose will depend on the relative heights of the practitioner and the client (see Fig. 8.1).

Technique

Work bilaterally with soft fists or elbows, sinking and then taking up a line of tension into the mid-belly of the trapezius. Carry the line of tension toward the trapezius attachments at the acromial processes (Fig. 8.1). Repeat 2–3 times.

Figure 8.1
Seated release of the trapezius.

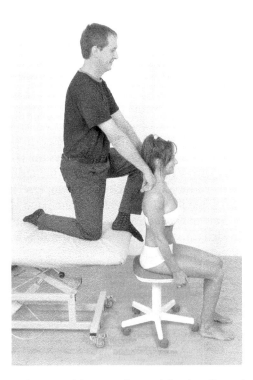

Repeat this procedure while the client drops their head forward and (slowly) rotates their head from one side to the other. Offer increased resistance to the contralateral side to the rotation (Fig. 8.2).

Have the client return their head to horizontal. Apply the same bilateral contact and then direct the line of tension toward the root of the spine of the scapula – inferior and only slightly lateral (Fig. 8.3). Repeat 2–3 times and have the client start to drop their head forward to increase the effect on the levator scapula.

Figure 8.2
Release of the trapezius in seated position with active client movement.

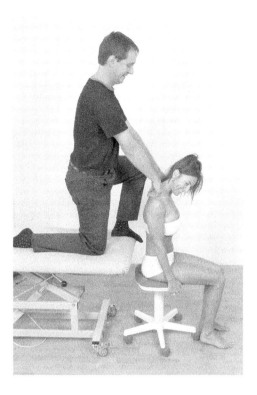

Figure 8.3
Seated release for levator scapula. Here the release is advanced, with the neck in flexion and the levator on active stretch.

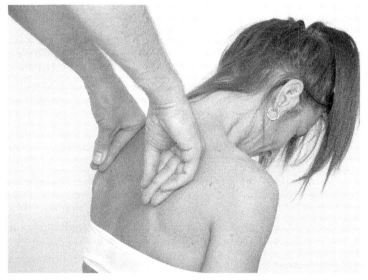

Work parallel to the spine by dragging down the erectors from superior to inferior. Start by focusing on the area of C7–T1, a notorious zone of stiffness, pain and dysfunction. The client curls forward and the contact is carried inferior, staying over the top of the erectors, down as far as the lumbosacral region (Fig. 8.4). A similar approach can be made more laterally on a line that runs along the vertebral border of the scapula and then onto the posterior angle of the ribs.

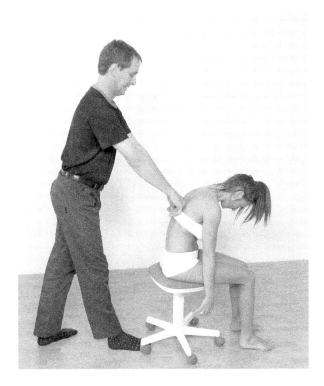

Figure 8.4
Seated release of erectors and thoracolumbar fascia.

Movement

To be effective these releases require a high degree of coordination and participation on the part of the client. The position requires both stabilization in the gravitational field and a client-controlled myofascial elongation – eccentric contraction of the thoracic and lumbar extensors – during the flexion phase of the release. Instruction on how to do this is essential. The movements must be supported through the feet and legs ... then have them push back from the whole of the feet into the point of contact rather than simply fold forward at the hips. Ask for them to explore this connection – they push back from their feet, which in turn are reaching deliberately through the floor with a specific sense of opening and direction. The body is curving (over a big beach ball is a useful image) while the point of contact is isolated and worked back into the pressure. Both people will be breathing easily if this is done well.

This is all worth persevering with. The initial efforts may be clumsy from both parties but in time this coordinated approach will click and the back will release beautifully in a way that prone work cannot even approach. This is integration – structure and coordination supporting change in each other.

Comments

The upper trapezius and levator scapula are tonic muscles that will often become overactive. Tension in this region can easily escalate to painful levels during times of emotional stress, prolonged lack of adequate postural support (working on a computer keyboard or when driving are common examples) or overexertion while giving bodywork treatments! Chronic hypertonicity will in turn overwhelm the lower scapula stabilizers and lead to other problems at the glenohumeral joint, cervical spine and occipital base. Tension headaches that originate in tight trapezius muscles are common. Getting release here is essential prior to any work on deeper cervical muscles, the suboccipital triangle or even the intracranial membranes.

PRONE BACK WORK – UPPER

Client

Prone with the lumbars stabilized at neutral with a pillow if there is hyperlordosis. A face cradle of some kind may be useful. Some people find these block the sinuses in which case turning the head to one side is quite acceptable.

Therapist

Initially standing at the head of the table. It will usually be necessary to move to one side of the table to treat the lumbar and lumbosacral regions.

Technique

1. Work bilaterally and use both hands in the soft fist position to make broad contact with the upper fibers of the mid trapezius in the region of C7–T1. Sink in a posterior inferior direction and once the tissue is well engaged, take up a line of tension and move further inferior (Fig. 8.5). A limitation will be reached when the therapist is fully extended and cannot go any further. At this point go to one side of the table and continue, across the thoracolumbar fascia and onto the sacrum.

Figure 8.5
Prone release of the superficial thoracic myofasciae.

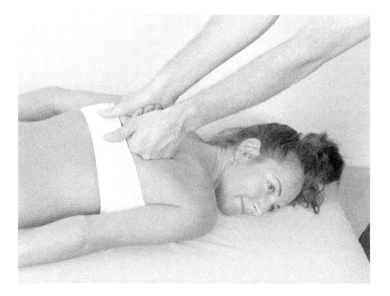

2. Work unilaterally. Use the blunt surface of the ulna just distal from the olecranon process to make contact with the trapezius at the same level as for the previous release. Sink on a line that is specifically directed at the area of the lamina groove and take up a line of tension in an inferior direction (Fig. 8.6). The goal is to work at the level of the trapezius and, on subsequent passes, the serratus posterior superior, splenius capitis, semispinalis cervicis and thoracis, and spinalis thoracis. Work as far as the mid to lower thoracic region and then repeat on the other side.

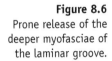

Figure 8.6
Prone release of the deeper myofasciae of the laminar groove.

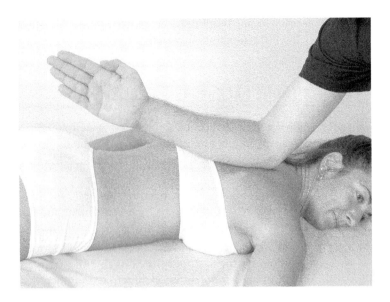

3. The contact is lateral to the previous technique. Treat in a similar manner the area of the longissimus thoracis (the most obviously rounded of the erectors) and the tissue immediately lateral to it as far as the mid to lower thoracic region. This can easily be done with the broad contact of the elbow. Repeat on the other side (Fig. 8.7).

Figure 8.7
Prone release of the longissimus thoracis region. Fingers shown here for photographic convenience – elbow might be better.

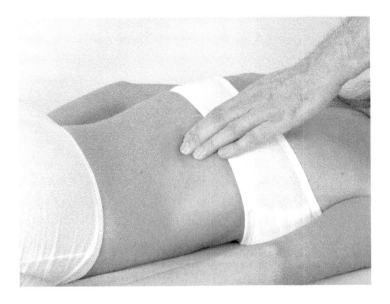

4. The contact is lateral to the previous technique. Treat the area of the iliocostalis thoracis and cervicis. Orient to these by locating the posterior angle of the ribs. There is less depth to the soft tissue here and the ribs will be easily located. Keep the angle at 15–25° so that the ribs are not displaced by too much direct vertical force (Fig. 8.8). Repeat on the other side.

Figure 8.8
Using the knuckles to apply MFR to the posterior angle of the ribs. This can be done with an elbow, fingers or knuckles.

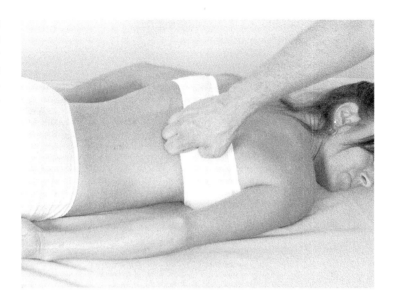

Movement

During the proximal portion of the last three releases, ask for the client to lift their head and rotate it to the opposite side. This can be guided with a broad contact through the palm of the non-treating hand. The eyes should be open and there is a deliberate sense of lengthening the neck as it rotates – a kind of 'uncorkscrewing' motion.

During any or all of the contacts, the client can be coached to direct their awareness to the points of contact with their breath. This is especially useful during releases 3 and 4 when the periosteum of the ribs can be engaged. Done well (shallow angle and slow speed), this provides wonderful stimulation to the nervous system. There can be many spontaneous releasing-type breaths as this work proceeds. The rib cage feels softer and becomes much more responsive to the inner motion of the breath as well as the pressure of the therapist.

Comments

This sequence of releases will greatly decrease stiffness in the thoracic spine and the posterior rib cage. Releasing the deeper muscles that cross from here to the neck will enable much greater continuity of spinal motion during cervical rotation. C7–T1 will be noticeably more responsive. The upper four thoracic vertebrae can then begin to join in on that cervical motion, making the entire rotational movement more coordinated and fluid.

Asthmatics will find the pliancy in the ribs helpful and even joyful. People who have had open heart surgeries, lobectomies and other thoracic surgeries will find that these releases restore space, movement and sensation to an area that may otherwise simply shrivel up and close off for life.

PRONE BACK WORK – LOWER

Client

Prone with the lumbars stabilized at neutral with a pillow if there is hyperlordosis. The feet are either off the end of the table or bolstered so as to allow for some dorsiflexion.

Therapist

Standing to the side of the table and facing towards the feet at the level of the client's waistline.

Technique

1. Work unilaterally. Use a blunt elbow to make a contact in the laminar groove at the level of T12 (Fig. 8.9). Once the tissue is engaged, add a line of tension in an inferior direction. The contact is focused at the surface (posterior layer of thoracolumbar fascia and latissimus dorsi) as well as the mid-layer muscles (longissimus and spinalis thoracis).

Figure 8.9
Prone release of the lumbar portion of the posterior layer of thoracolumbar fascia.

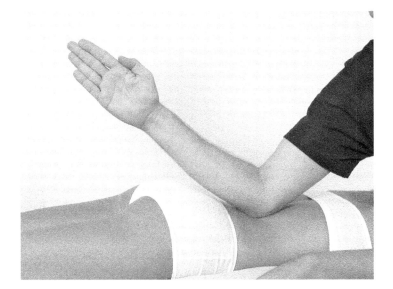

2. Continue working unilaterally. Sink slowly to make a contact through the surface and mid-layer muscles into the deeper multifidus. Once this level is contacted, develop a line of tension in an inferior direction that can then be carried across onto the sacrum (Fig. 8.10). The multifidus tendon blends with

Figure 8.10
Prone release of the deeper lumbar myofasciae.

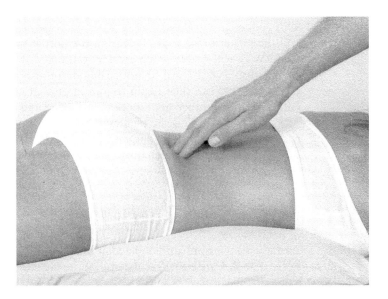

the fascia associated with the sacrotuberous and long dorsal sacroiliac ligament. Stable fingers may provide more precise palpation and engagement with the distal aspects of this contact than the elbow.

3. Find the transverse process of L5. This is done by first finding the more easily palpated process of L4, which is generally adjacent to the top of the iliac crest (and usually much deeper in the tissue than expected). Use a supported thumb to palpate the area immediately inferior to the L5 process. Locate the small zone of soft tissue between the iliac crest and the vertebra. There is rarely room to put a line of tension into the soft tissue so generally, just maintain the slow sinking intention (Fig. 8.11). Repeat on the other side.

Figure 8.11
MFR of the multifidus and associated fascia.

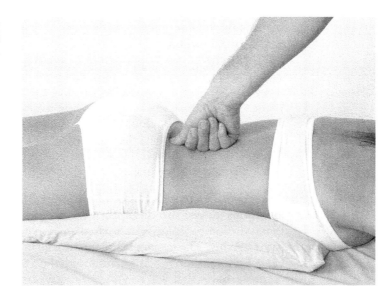

4. Use a broad elbow, soft fist or well-supported fingers to engage the soft tissues over the posterior angle of the lower ribs (Fig. 8.12). This will affect the

Figure 8.12
MFR to the lateral portions of the thoracolumbar fascia.

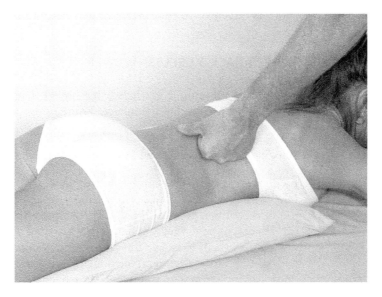

thoracolumbar fascia, serratus posterior inferior, iliocostalis thoracis and lumborum. Carry the line of tension off the ribs and into the waistline. Subsequent passes can go more deeply to contact the anterior layer of the thoracolumbar fascia, transversus abdominis aponeurosis and quadratus lumborum.

Movement

When the latissimus dorsi and thoracolumbar fascia are contacted, the client can slowly slide their ipsilateral arm along the table (abduction). As a preparatory movement, ask for the fingers to spread open and generate a pleasant feeling of stretch in the palmar surface of the hand, with direction – 'Slide your arm slowly toward the wall/picture/vase/painting/the door you came in through'.

The ipsilateral leg can also be encouraged to open. First lift the toes, which will put a light stretch in the plantar fascia. Then lengthen through the heel into deliberate but unforced dorsiflexion. This creates a beautiful sense of opening in two directions.

With the deeper myofascia – multifidus, anterior thoracolumbar fascia – the movement can be focused more locally. Being careful not to overpressure, have the client push a specific vertebra back against the contact but without using a pelvic tilt. The range is small: 2–3 cm. Finding this degree of coordination requires time and must be done after the superficial spinal erectors are eased and released. 'First find this point of contact in your awareness ... slowly ... easy ... no rush ... now push this specific vertebra back into my elbow' as an example. This can also be done against bilateral pressure.

Comments

The lower spinal erectors are tonic muscles that often overpower the underlying multifidus muscle and this in turn contributes to a loss of dynamic stabilization in the lumbar spine. Overexcited erectors and sleepy multifidus lead to lumbar instability. The good news is that the chances of altering this state are high as the thoracolumbar fascia and multifidus triangle are richly innervated with sensory fibers that will respond to the types of stimulation our elbows, fingers and thumbs can provide here. Direct technique MFR, with its pressure, shearing forces and associated coordinated movements, will lower tone, reduce pain, increase pleasant sensations and reawaken proprioception. Clearly, then, there are advantages to including these aspects of release in conjunction with any endeavor to educate about new neuromuscular coordination.

DEEPER BACK MUSCLES – LOWER

Client

Seated with attention to the hips being higher than the knees, feet slightly forward of the knees and well connected to the ground. The client supports their back via their feet and legs.

Therapist

Standing behind the client and working bilaterally into the thoracolumbar fascia.

Technique

Identify areas of stiffness in the lumbar spine by palpation or motion testing. Use well-supported thumbs or fingertips to engage bilaterally in the tissues on top of the lamina groove (Fig. 8.13). The pressure is firm and anterior. Have the client connect very deliberately with their feet by pushing into them slightly. Ask them to isolate the points of pressure against their spine and then push to them from their feet, introducing lumbar flexion into a very local zone only. Encourage them to isolate the specific segment on which you are maintaining the pressure. Once it is isolated, have the direction reversed so that now the segment is going anterior (local extension without pelvic tilt) while there is still deliberate connection through to the ground via the feet.

Figure 8.13
Increasing spinal stability via pressure into the myofasciae, combined with coordinated movement. Lumbar section.

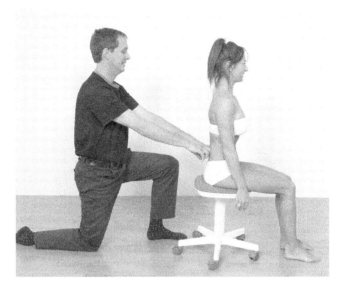

Movement

With this release, the movement and the technique are inseparable. This is really about coordination done in a very precise manner. The feet should be encouraged to open and feel fully into the floor ... through the floor. This sensation can be maintained throughout all phases of the contact. The range of movement in the lumbar vertebrae is small – approximately 3 cm.

Comments

There are a number of key elements to be considered here. First, the lower spinal erectors need to be released through either the broad seated work or the prone position releases described above. Next, the attention must stay on the motion being at a local level so that the multifidus are activating through precise eccentric and concentric contractions rather than engaging the erector muscles. Watch for the pelvis initiating the movement or the whole lumbar region moving at once – this will be the erectors at work. Check to see if the neck or thoracic spine attempts to do all of the movement and bypass the local site of contact. Direct the attention back to the contact points if they do. This whole process takes time to master and is incredibly useful when it has been.

DEEPER BACK MUSCLES – UPPER

Client

Seated as for above with the hands on the wall at the level of the shoulders.

Therapist

As for above.

Technique

Identify areas of stiffness in the thoracic spine by palpation or motion testing. Use well-supported thumbs or fingertips to engage in the tissues on top of the lamina groove. The pressure is firm, without overexertion, and anterior. Have the client connect very deliberately with their hands by reaching into them slightly. The hands are encouraged to spread broadly against the wall so the contact is as universal as possible (Fig. 8.14). Use this deliberate contact through the hands to initiate the movement. Keep the same degree of connection throughout the microflexion and extension movements.

Figure 8.14
Increasing spinal stability via pressure into the myofasciae, combined with coordinated movement. Thoracic section.

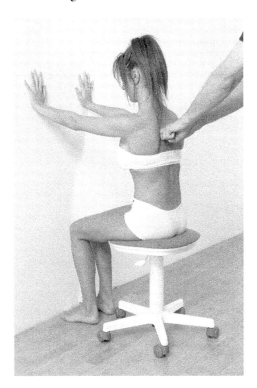

Movement

Direct awareness to the sensations of the hands engaged with the wall. This will automatically reduce the amount of tension in the pectoralis major and allow the lower scapula stabilizers to activate instead. Once the hands are clearly in awareness then add a return to the contact of the feet so the movement is guided from both the floor and the wall.

Comments

This approach to releasing and activating the smaller muscles of the upper back is best after the bigger, broader ones have been addressed. The nervous system 'noise' associated with tight upper trapezius, levator scapula and, sometimes, the upper erector muscles must be reduced before this coordination will work. Once the deeper multifidus are activated, the return of thoracic extension and stability will be immediate. Chronic facet joint irritations associated with instability will often resolve after this release.

THE TRUNK – SIDES

LATISSIMUS DORSI, THORACOLUMBAR FASCIA, EXTERNAL AND INTERNAL OBLIQUES

Client

Sidelying, head supported by a pillow. Hips at 45° of flexion. Knees at 35° of flexion.

Therapist   Standing behind the client at hip level.

Technique   **1.** Use a soft fist, stable fingers or elbow to contact the soft tissues in the waist-line, at the midline of the coronal plane. Sink medially towards the table and engage the first layers of resistance (Fig. 8.15). Pause while the person's aware-ness comes to meet the contact. This will often be followed by sensations of melting associated with a therapeutic breath. Next, put a line of tension in a posterior direction until the PSIS is contacted.

Figure 8.15
MFR to the superficial portion of the waistline.

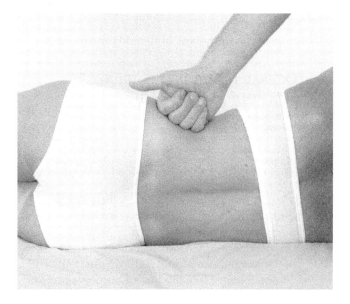

2. Repeat this process with attention to the deeper, underlying internal oblique and iliocostalis lumborum tendons. Engage the tissue and release in the same direction as above (Fig. 8.16).

Figure 8.16
MFR to the deeper structures of the waistline.

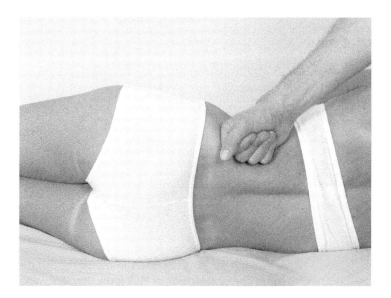

Movement

The client abducts and externally rotates the ipsilateral arm toward a specific location and also steps down deliberately through into the heel of the ipsilateral leg (knee and hip extension with ankle dorsiflexion).

Direct the inhalation toward the point of contact.

Comments

This is deeper work than the iliac crest release in the lower extremities chapter. Spend more time sinking into the layers of tissue before engaging a line of tension. This is a potent site for neurofascial release due to the large number of sensory fibers. Many broad tendons converge here with the thoracolumbar fascia. Sometimes deep pressure can be maintained here for several minutes. Monitor the client's breathing response, tonus changes and facial affect to confirm the usefulness of the longer contact.

LATERAL ASPECT OF THE TRUNK

Client

Sidelying, head supported by a pillow. Hips at 45° of flexion. Knees at 35° of flexion. The ipsilateral arm is abducted over the head with the palm of the hand resting either on the head or on the pillow above it.

Therapist

Standing behind the client at the level of the hips and facing toward the head.

Technique

1. Use the fingerpads to engage the tissue over the 11th rib (or 12th if it can be readily palpated). Sink through to the level of the rib so that both the overlying soft tissues and the periosteum are being contacted (Fig. 8.17). Develop a superior line of tension that takes in the next two ribs, the anterior fibers of the latissimus dorsi and serratus posterior inferior as well as the external oblique. Next, carry the line of tension posteriorly into the lateral margins of the thoracolumbar fascia.

Figure 8.17
MFR to the lower lateral ribs.

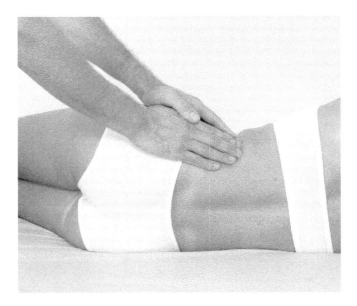

2. Reposition the fingerpads to the area of the 8th rib (Fig. 8.18). There will often be room for both hands at this level. Repeat a similar process of engagement and line of tension. This will take in the external oblique, lower sections of the serratus anterior and the edge of the latissimus dorsi. The underlying external intercostal muscle can also be affected in this way.

Figure 8.18
MFR to the mid-lateral ribs.

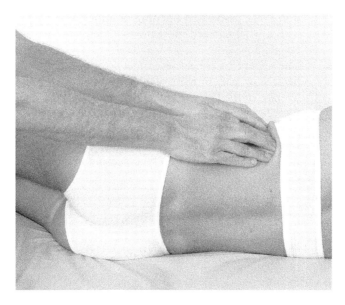

3. Reposition the fingerpads over the 5th rib (Fig. 8.19). Sink through to the level of the rib so that both the covering soft tissues and the periosteum are being contacted. Develop a superior line of tension that takes in the next 2–3 ribs. This superior movement will terminate in the upper portion of the axilla.

Figure 8.19
MFR to the upper rib cage and axillary fascia.

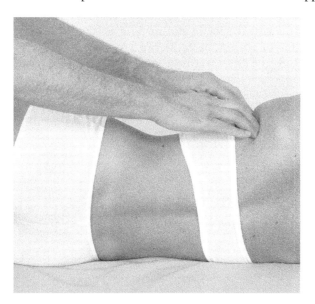

Movement

The ipsilateral arm is in abduction with elbow flexion to at least 90°. The hand is then able to rest on the side of the head or on the pillow superior to it. Encourage deliberate contact into the whole hand, not just the heel. During any of the preceding contacts the client can be encouraged to lengthen through the humerus and transmit the weight into the hand. This is a closed chain movement that will activate more of the proprioception in the arm. Another, open chain movement is to have the client reach over their head while externally rotating the elbow (toward the ceiling). This will lengthen the latissimus dorsi. The associated opening of either movement approach can be supported with a synchronized inbreath that facilitates increased motion in the ribs.

Comments

The upper ribs are always tender so taking things slowly will get the best results here. Slow, patient work will be rewarded with significant changes in the responsiveness of the ribs to breathing, which is useful for asthma and other respiratory disorders. The release can contribute to activation of the serratus anterior – via proprioceptive stimulation – with associated scapula stabilization. Work this whole lateral line for release of a fixed and exaggerated thoracic kyphosis. The ribs in the axilla will often be especially stiff and fixed with this pattern.

THE TRUNK – SUPERFICIAL FRONT

RECTUS ABDOMINIS AND SHEATH

Client

Supine.

Therapist

Standing at the client's side at the level of the pelvis, facing toward the head.

Technique

1. Have the client momentarily lift their head towards the ceiling to activate the rectus abdominis. Use this action to locate the lateral aspects of the rectus sheath approximately 2 cm above the pubis. Work bilaterally with the hands angled onto the contact at 45°. Sink vertically into the soft tissue immediately lateral to the rectus sheath. Engage the first distinct layer of tension and put a line of tension in a superior and medial direction. Slowly 'scoop' under the sheath while carrying the line of tension superiorly (Fig. 8.20). Repeat this approach incrementally up to the costal arch.

Figure 8.20
MFR to the rectus sheath.

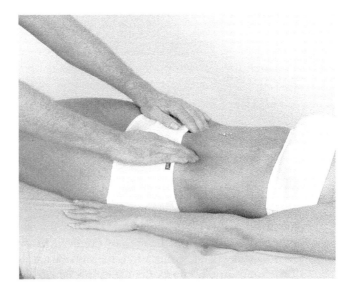

2. Work bilaterally. At the costal arch, position the fingers so that the same superior and medial line of tension can be employed. This means following the shape of the arch (Fig. 8.21). The contact is deliberately engaging both the overlying soft tissue as well as the underlying cartilage. Make a series of contacts along the inferior surface of the cartilage as well as the anterior. The heels of the hands can rest lightly on the abdominal wall to facilitate entry into the inferior aspect.

Figure 8.21
MFR to the costal arch and associated myofasciae.

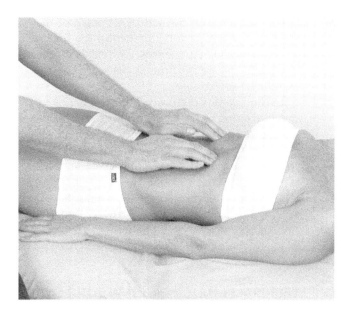

3. Work bilaterally. Position the fingerpads onto the costal cartilage of the 7th ribs (Fig. 8.22). Engage through the rectus abdominis onto the cartilage and then take up a superior line of tension. Carry these lines of tension up to at least the 5th costal cartilages. With women, these lines will have to stay on top of the sternum. With men, they can of course be more lateral.

Figure 8.22
MFR to the upper fibers of rectus abdominis.

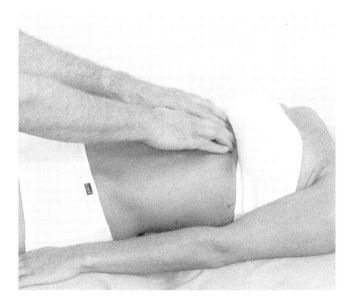

Movement

The myofascial release of the rectus sheath and associated structures can be augmented with synchronized inhalation that facilitates increased motion in the ribs. 'Imagine you are breathing through the skin here right into my fingers.' Attention should be given to ensuring that the lumbar spine does not go into lordosis during the inbreath. This can be discouraged by directing the breath towards the sides and back.

Comments

The rectus sheath is formed by a branch of the overlying external abdominal oblique aponeurosis and a branch of the underlying aponeurosis of the transversus abdominis. Aponeuroses are richly innervated with fascial sensory fibers. Myofascial release into the fascial seams on the lateral margins of the sheath has a broad effect.

Tension in this region can be closely linked to chronic anxiety states that involve fixating into a whole body flexion pattern. Psychologic states give birth to deep tensions in the anterior aspect of the trunk which can prevent full excursion of the ribs during inhalation. At its most extreme, this flexion fixation can result in the classic sunken chest, a hallmark of the so-called posture of defeat. Tensions through the rectus abdominis will also inhibit the activity of the underlying transversus abdominis. Successful core stabilization requires sustained proprioceptive access to the underlying transversus abdominis and internal oblique muscles. The releases described here will be enormously useful in awakening that self-awareness.

PECTORALIS MAJOR AND INVESTING LAYER OF PECTORALIS MINOR

Client

Supine.

Therapist

Standing at the client's side at the level of the waistline, facing toward the head. For the first technique, stand to the contralateral side.

Technique

1. Work unilaterally. Use the fingerpads of both hands to engage the soft tissue over the body of the sternum, from just superior to the xyphoid process (Fig. 8.23). Work through the overlying soft tissues to the level of the sternum. Develop a line of tension in the direction of the coracoid process. Initially, the contact is largely tendon, ligament, cartilage and bone. The depth of soft tissue increases as the bulk of the pectoralis major is encountered. An initial pass will be more surface than subsequent ones. By the third pass the underlying investing layer of fascia will be contacted with a clear sense of the ribs as well.
2. Work unilaterally. Reposition the hands so that the upper aspects of the pectoralis major are engaged (Fig. 8.24). Start again at the sternum and carry the line of tension across to the coracoid process. Contact the inferior aspect of the clavicle. The initial contact will be at the surface but subsequent ones will engage the deeper investing layers of pectoralis minor and subclavius fasciae.
3. Work unilaterally. Use the pads of the fingers of one hand to engage the soft tissue just medial to the coracoid process (Fig. 8.25). Put a line of tension across the process in a superior lateral direction. Keep the tension in place on the anterior surface of the process while the client externally rotates and abducts their arm.

Figure 8.23
MFR to the pectoralis
major and investing fascia.

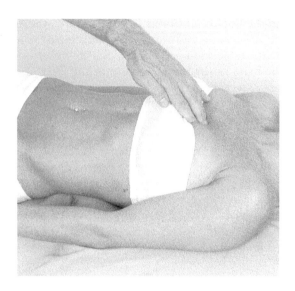

Figure 8.24
MFR to the pectoralis
minor and subclavius
muscles.

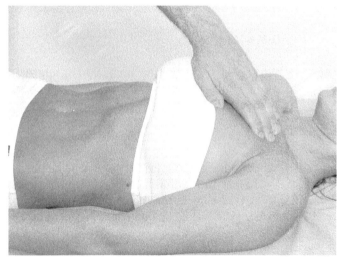

Figure 8.25
Release of the tendons at
the coracoid process with
active client movement.

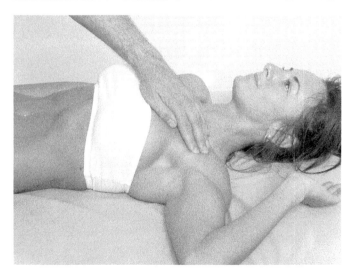

Movement

While the line of tension is carried towards the coracoid process, the client slowly abducts the ipsilateral arm. 'Reach past your head by sliding your arm across the table and opening your fingers towards the wall.'

The hand of the ipsilateral arm is initially resting on the abdomen. While the upper section of the pectoralis major is being worked, the client introduces slow external rotation of that arm until the dorsum of the hand is resting on the table. Simultaneously, during the external rotation, they rotate their head and neck away to the contralateral side: 'Roll your head and look towards the ceiling back over your shoulder'.

With a sustained and firm line of tension on the coracoid process (without any painful overpressure) the client makes small or even micro movements of abduction and adduction at the shoulder so the tissues overlying the bone are put on a series of slight stretches. A longer 'macro' motion of the arm into abduction is also possible.

THE TRUNK – DEEP FRONT

ADVANCED PSOAS

Client

Supine with the knees and hips both at approximately 90° of flexion. This requires a suitable stool or chair placed on the table, a large firm bolster or a number of pillows.

Therapist

Standing to one side at the level of the hips.

Technique

1. Work unilaterally. Draw an imaginary line between the ASIS and the umbilicus. Contact the abdominal wall at a point on that line halfway between the ASIS and the edge of the rectus sheath (Fig. 8.26). Use the pads of the fingers of either both hands or one hand supported by the other to sink posteriorly

Figure 8.26
Advanced release of the psoas – client passive.

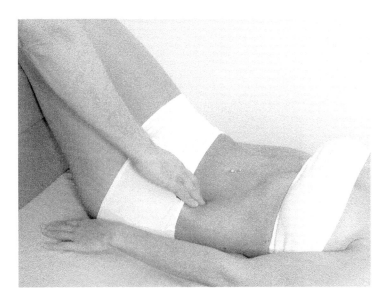

until the first barrier to further motion is encountered. Wait until the barrier releases and follow the release down into the visceral cavity without any overpressure. The direction continues to be largely posterior with 10–15° of medial angle toward the spine added. Engage the next barrier and wait for softening. Proceed in this mindful manner until the anterior fibers of the psoas are contacted. This may take up to 5 minutes.

2. Work unilaterally. Continue the process from above until the psoas sheath is felt to release and its deeper fibers can be contacted. Sometimes the anterior lateral aspect of the lumbar vertebrae can be felt although this is not essential for the release to be effective. The client is directed to push the contralateral leg down onto the stool (calf makes increased contact). While this moderate movement is engaged, pick the ipsilateral leg up from behind the knee and introduce some small rotational movements at the hip while verbally encouraging the client to let the hip muscles relax (Fig. 8.27). The effect of this will be to have the abdominal wall drop into the table, a hallmark of successful release of the deep psoas.

Figure 8.27
Advanced release of the psoas with active client movement.

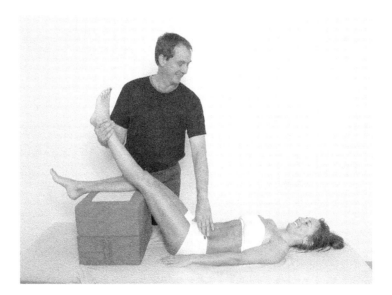

Movement

As described above for part 2. When the entry into the psoas is slow and mindful, there should be no muscle guarding at all. The hip and abdominal muscles will then easily accommodate the movement introduced by the therapist at the hip. Once the movement is successful in a small range it can be extended into larger rotations, flexion, extension, abduction and adduction. Bring the client's attention to the 'internal massage' of the hip joint that the movement will create. This can quickly start to feel very pleasurable.

Comments

Many psoases, and their accompanying person, have been traumatized by the local disintegrative manual therapist via work that goes too deeply and quickly. Think of the psoas as being at the literal *and* metaphoric core of a person's being. This will shift the intention from stretching a pesky tight rubber band to one of curiosity about how the natives of the deep abdominal region are communicating with each other and the outside world; this is much more respectful. Releasing the psoas is just as delicious and relaxing as getting a hypervigilant suboccipital region to release and equally as important in terms of the effect on the ANS.

THE RESPIRATORY DIAPHRAGM

Client

Supine with the legs supported as for the psoas release above.

Therapist

Standing beside the client at the level of diaphragm and treating the contralateral side.

Technique

Locate the xyphoid and the costal arch. Using the fingers, sink posteriorly just medial to the xyphoid and inferior to the costal arch (Fig. 8.28). Wait for an initial softening before directing the contact up under the arch (superior). A lateral line of tension can then be introduced. This is not a continuous movement but a series of contacts that work in increments towards the floating ribs.

Figure 8.28
MFR to the respiratory diaphragm.

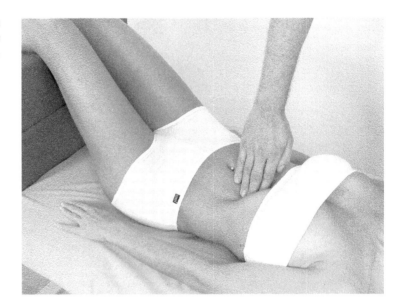

Movement

The client's awareness will naturally go to the breathing. Increased attention to a deliberate but unforced exhalation, with a prolonged preinspiration phase (pause before inhalation), will assist in the release process. 'Let the ribs collapse like a bag of bones on the exhale.'

Comments

Anxiety states will often include significant involvement of the superficial and deep front of the trunk respiratory muscles. This high-tone, apprehensive state contributes to a significant postural pattern that includes a loss of full excursion of the ribs during inhalation. Other associated breathing patterns can include chronic hyperventilation with a non-exerted respiratory rhythm of 16 cycles a minute or above. With chronic hyperventilation there is generally no preinspiration phase at all. The effect of this is that the resting, non-exerted breath becomes a kind of panting. I see and hear this panting often with clients who are in pain when they come for work, as well as in cases of undiagnosed subclinical, and diagnosed, anxiety states. The general effect of panting is to create a reduction in CO_2 which in turn will generate an excitement of the SNS. This is the classic fight or flight physiologic state occurring when there is nothing in the environment actually posing a threat to the organism's survival.

What makes anxiety states so destructive is that all this survival mode stuff, designed for the short haul only, happens when in fact there is no saber-toothed tiger at the door of our cave at all. Yet through a complex process in which images arise in the mind and the body reacts as if the images are real, the same unpleasant and self-perpetuating physiologic states will develop. In turn, the unpleasant physiologic state confirms that the images we generated are in fact associated with real 'bad stuff' and the loop is complete.

Interrupting this cycle – evident to some extent in the majority of my clients and a major contributor to them being disoriented in time and space – is actually very simple and incredibly useful. The techniques described so far in this section for the anterior trunk, both deep and superficial, will have a major impact on the breathing. Coupled with the educational approach described below, the client can leave with a set of strategies for further developing breathing that supports a happy, satisfying and expressive life.

Breathing releases are not just about the ribs or only for people with respiratory disorders like asthma. Norbet Weiner observed that 'We are not stuff that abides but patterns that perpetuate themselves'. Nowhere is this more evident than in the breath. As already mentioned, patterns of bodily tension associated with psychophysical armoring, the physical mediation of emotion and unresolved shock trauma all find expression in the breath. Physical insults of all kinds usually involve a modification of the breath.

The breath is a barometer. It tells us a lot more about a person than simply what the motion in the ribs is. A friendly non-invasive contact to any part of a person that leads to feelings of release, decompression and well-being will be expressed via an accompanying therapeutic breath. This is a spontaneous full breath with a complete, relaxed exhalation followed by an unforced prolonged preinspiration phase. These therapeutic breaths occur frequently in integrative somatics sessions (rarely, if at all, at the office of the disintegrative manual therapist, except perhaps when leaving) and are a good indicator that the work is proceeding well.

A classification system can be proposed for two basic respiratory patterns.

1. *Expiration fixed.* This is characterized by a shortness in the anterior myofascia of the trunk. It is associated with exaggerated thoracic kyphosis, hypertonic pectoralis, upper trapezius, subscapularis and biceps muscles as well as tension at the suboccipital triangle. There is adduction of the extremities. The lumbar spine can be in neutral, hyperlordosis or kyphosis.

2. *Inspiration fixed.* With this pattern the emphasis is on the inbreath and the ribs will be perpetually elevated. The erector muscles of the spine will be hypertonic, normal thoracic kyphosis will be diminished, with thoracic lordosis in extreme cases. The extremities will be in abduction with tensions in the deep hip rotators, infraspinatus and triceps. The lumbar spine is often kyphotic with a posterior pelvis and the sacrum in a locked and counternutated position.

FREEING THE BREATHING – A FUNCTIONAL APPROACH #1

Client

Supine with the knees supported on pillows, bolsters, etc. to give approximately 45° of hip flexion.

Therapist

Standing at the client's side at the level of the shoulder and angled onto their body at 45° – medial and inferior. The angles of movement of the therapist's body during the release will match the movement of the ribs during exhalation: inferior, medial and posterior.

Technique

Place your hands as shown in Figure 8.29. Try to make the contact as broad as possible, not just at the thenar and hyperthenar eminences. Ask the client for an exaggerated inhalation while providing firm pressure through the hands. This will give good proprioceptive awareness of the position of the ribs.

During exhalation, exaggerate the three motions – inferior, medial and posterior – while verbally encouraging the client to allow for the complete release of air. Maintain the same moderate three-dimensional resistance while the client again inhales. Take the ribs into an exaggerated exhale once more. A third cycle of inhalation/exhalation can be used; it is useful to have this third breath cycle 'cut short' by coaching the client to take a smaller inbreath than the previous two prior to once again exaggerating the exhalation.

Figure 8.29
Functional release for the ribs.

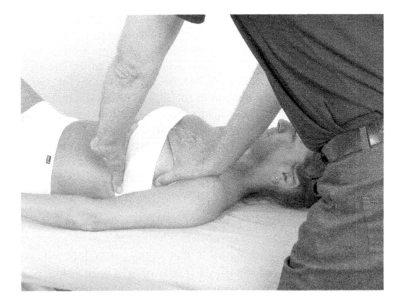

Movement

With all the functional techniques, movement is central to the process of release and cannot be described separately from it.

It is worth reinforcing the spatial attitude of the therapist as this is essential to the successful transmission of the releasing forces. The key to efficient lengthening movement is direction (see p43) which gives rise to good coordination. To deliver a good contact here, first connect with the feet as fully engaging with the floor; through it even. Then the hands make the same opening contact into the client's body; the shoulders will automatically drop and the scapula stabilize once these two directions are felt. It is sensory, not conceptual. Once the movement commences, it feels more like a tai chi 'push hands' motion – circular, lengthening, without effort – rather than a push-up being done on the client's chest.

When this type of contact is made, our bodies can model the kind of connected, embodied state that we are guiding our clients towards rediscovering. Looking for a reduction of overexertion from your client? Try modeling it as you work and see how a reciprocal state will quickly develop. Try thinking of touch as a way of saying hello, of being curious, rather than the more medical 'I'm fixing this broken thingy here with my highly trained manipulation'.

Comments

Allow time for 'self sensing' after the release cycle is complete. For many people this is where the real change occurs as the body reawakens to its potentials for ease and decompression. Spatial awareness is significantly altered by these releases. This can result in a sudden awareness of the various dynamics that have contributed to the loss of this organic well-being – the emotional undercurrents often surge to the surface. Don't be surprised or alarmed if there are tears, sobbing, groaning or other signs of emotions surfacing. These can occur while simultaneously encouraging the person to stay in touch with their breath and their surroundings. Kindly bring attention back to their sensation; of the breath; of their weight on the table; the color of the walls. It can be very empowering to discover that strong emotions can be experienced without going into disconnected, disembodied states of catharsis. This is not psychotherapy but simply skillful body therapy. It is my observation that unless the client has an underlying psychiatric disorder – psychosis or schizophrenia, for example – then the emotions that arise in somatic therapy are integrated by the client themselves both on the table and in the days following the session.

FREEING THE BREATH #2

Client

Supine with the knees supported on pillows, bolsters, etc. to give approximately 45° of hip flexion.

Therapist

Standing at the client's side at the level of the shoulder and angled onto their body at 45° – medial and inferior. The angles of movement of the therapist's body during the release will match the movement of the ribs during exhalation: inferior, medial and posterior.

Technique

Place your upper hand as shown in Figure 8.30. The hand on the posterior surface is across the scapula with the heel just medial to the humeral head and the fingers at the vertebral border, mirroring the direction of the upper hand.

Ask the client for an exaggerated inhalation while providing moderate resistance to the movement of the ribs and shoulder. Exaggerate the exhalation by rolling the shoulder from lateral to medial and posterior to anterior. The posterior hand protracts the scapula. Maintain the moderate three-dimensional resistance while the client again inhales. Create an exaggerated exhale, past the client's normal endpoint for the rib motion. Hold the compression momentarily and verbally encourage full relaxation. On the third cycle of inhalation/exhalation, do the 'cut short' version rather than another full inhalation.

Figure 8.30
Functional release for the
upper ribs and pectoralis
minor.

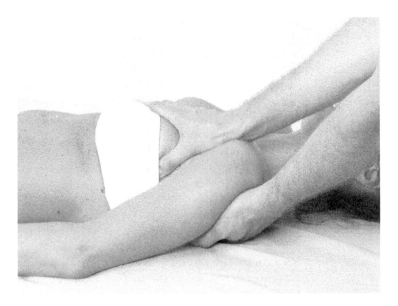

Movement   As for above. The shorter duration of the third inhale enables the sensations to stay fresh. Fresh, of course, means new and, in a sense, also unpredictable. Once the person senses the frequency and amplitude of the movements, they will start trying, generally without any conscious intent, to do them. This generates unwanted effort at a time when we are wanting to take over the work so they can let go.

Comments   As for above.

FREEING THE BREATH #3

Client   Sidelying.

Therapist   Standing behind the client at the level of the head and facing inferior and anterior. The therapist's position should reflect the need for the lines of movement that duplicate all the motions of the ribs. In particular, this release requires attention to the longitudinal movement and not just the medial.

Technique   **1.** Place your hands as shown in Figure 8.31a. The superior hand cups the shoulder girdle with the thumb resting on the scapula and fingers resting on the clavicle. The inferior hand is resting into the axilla with the web of the hand crossing the rib cage at the level of R3. The client takes a full inhalation against moderate resistance, with attention to the sides of the body responding to the breath. On the exhalation, depress the shoulder girdle and ribs in concert. The depressive motion is threefold – inferior, medial and slightly anterior. Repeat the cycle as per the previous releases.
2. Leave the superior hand in the same position as for #1. Move the inferior hand to R5 (Fig. 8.31b, c). Repeat the procedure.

Figure 8.31
(a) Functional release for shoulder girdle and upper ribs. The arm has been left in the abducted position to show the hand placement in the axilla.
(b) Second position for the sequence of releasing the shoulder girdle and the lateral aspect of the ribs. The arm is correctly positioned for this and the previous release.
(c) A posterior view showing the hand placement for the second position.

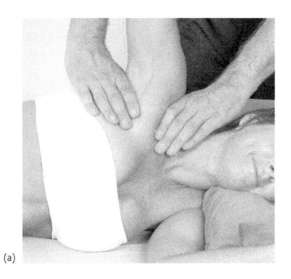

(a)

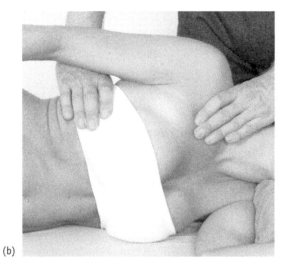

(b)

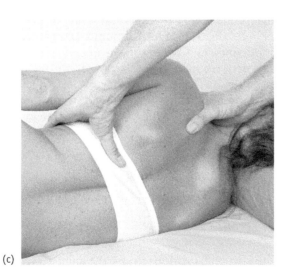

(c)

3. Move the superior hand off the shoulder girdle and onto the ribs in the axilla. The inferior hand is placed on the area of R9–10 (Fig. 8.32). Both hands work in concert to repeat the process of breathing in against resistance and so on.

Figure 8.32
Functional release of the lateral rib cage – both hands on the ribs.

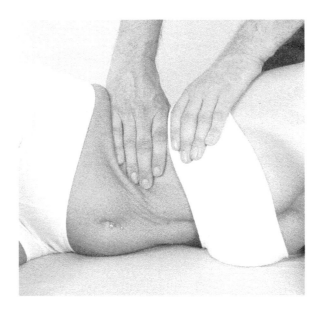

Movement

Keep the hand contacts as broad and soft as possible. Beware of any tendency to only compress the ribs medially. This is painful and can even dislodge the rib at the spine if the effort is too forceful and local.

Comments

Because there are a number of releases done in succession, the risk of acute hyperventilation must be considered. To avoid this, keep the pace slow and take breaks after each repositioning of the hands. Encourage normal, unforced breathing with slightly prolonged preinspiration during these breaks.

Functional techniques provide sudden shifts in sensations of pressure and range of motion. These serve to wake up the nervous system and provoke a rapid reevaluation of muscle tonus and fascial tensioning via the intrafascial smooth muscles. Changes to the underlying tonus of the gamma system, associated with emotional states expressed through the skeletal muscle, might well explain the surfacing of grief, sorrow and anger. While it may not be the therapist's intention to provoke these releases, nevertheless they will arise when the breath is released in this fashion. Strategies on how to respond to these states are given in Chapter 3.

PEDIATRIC SUPPLEMENT FOR THE TRUNK

SEATED BACK WORK

Client

Seated, with adaptations to suit the child's level of development.

Therapist   Adapted to suit the situation. The general guideline is to have a stable base of support and be above the points of contact so that the bodyweight can easily be directed into the work.

Technique   Work the back in the same manner as shown in the adult section. Here the child is shown on the table in a self-supported folded position (Fig. 8.33). Bolsters and pillows could be used to provide support.

Figure 8.33
Seated back work adapted
to the pediatric setting.

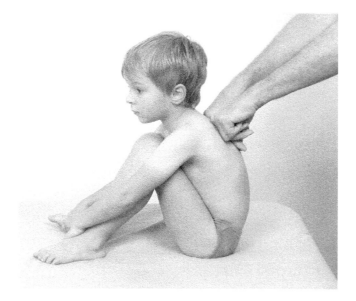

Movement   Must be adapted to suit the developmental stage of the child. Very often, there will be spontaneous unfocused movements – wriggling, squirming and so on. These can often be used to augment the MFR.

Comments   With the child, the back work is often about facilitating better extensor tone rather than reducing it. The work in the back is then done more quickly with less attention to sinking and melting. Stimulation replaces pacification. The need for this can frequently be observed where the trunk flexors are short and tight while the erectors are long and inactive. In these situations, treat the flexor tone first. Of course, the erectors might simply be hypertonic and need release. In this instance the tone in the back muscles is the primary restriction and can be approached first with more attention to a melting style.

Chapter 9
INTRAORAL TREATMENT

It would be fair to say that direct technique MFR in the mouth is potentially the most intrusive that there is. 'Potentially' is stressed here; work within the mouth can and should be highly relaxing.

For most of us there seem to be two extremes with the mouth – the joys of eating, talking, drinking and kissing contrasted with painful trips to the dentist, where one small point of pain can fill an entire nervous system universe. Approaching someone with a latex glove and the request to 'now just open your mouth' will generally be associated more with the latter experience than the former. A verbal introduction to what you are planning on doing is therefore highly recommended. An anatomy text, with the page for the jaw muscles marked in advance, can be brought out to show the muscles and bones of the region.

It has been my consistent observation that there is considerable local release, and then subsequent whole body relaxation, when intraoral work is done well. This occurs surprisingly rapidly. Do all the releases on one side and then give the client some time to explore the new sensations of ease, relaxation and space. The work then starts to speak for itself. One side feels like a palace; the other like a pigeon coop.

The broad effect is not surprising really, given the huge amount of sensory fibers in the mouth and lips.

FASCIAE OF MANDIBLE

Client Supine, with a few degrees of capital extension.

Therapist Seated on a stool at the head of the table and facing towards the feet.

Technique Work with the client's mouth slightly open. Use the first finger to apply moderate sinking pressure into the soft tissue just medial to the coronoid process (Fig. 9.1). The pad of the finger will contact the periosteum of the mandible while the tip will sink into the soft tissue that is the interior surface of the cheek (deep portion of masseter). After a response is felt (jaw drops open, tissue softens, stiffness in TMJ eases), release the pressure and reposition. Repeat the process of sinking and release. Work the vestibule of the mouth, all the way along the mandible from the TMJ to the frenulum of the lower lip.

Figure 9.1
Finger position for release of the fasciae of the mandible. This is about the halfway point for the series of contacts along the bony/fascial surface.

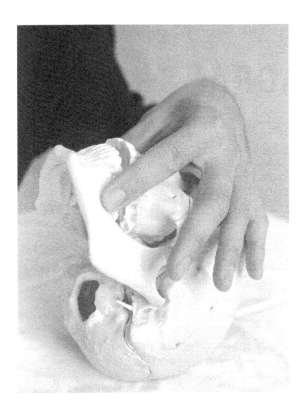

Movement

Once contact and release have occurred and the therapist's hand is withdrawn, the client will generally go on a 'search and feel' trip with their tongue. There is also often a great deal of jaw jiggling/yawning done in conjunction with this tongue journey. Allow time for this exploration of new space and, usually, a rapid reduction in stiffness in the TMJ.

Comments

This is one of the highest leverage sites in the body. The wide-ranging effects of this and the other intraoral releases are predictable. The suboccipital triangle and associated larger craniocervical muscles will release; the TMJ will decompress; the constrictor muscles in the throat will release; sinuses will clear; accessory breathing muscles (SCM and scalenes) will relax. Tongue placement, jaw position and swallowing can all be expected to improve.

FASCIAE OF MAXILLAE

Client

Supine, with a small amount of capital extension.

Therapist

Seated on a chair at around shoulder level and facing superiorly.

Technique

Essentially this is a mirror image of the release for the mandible. Commence from beneath the zygomatic arch and work incrementally to the frenulum of the upper lip (Fig. 9.2).

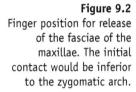

Figure 9.2
Finger position for release of the fasciae of the maxillae. The initial contact would be inferior to the zygomatic arch.

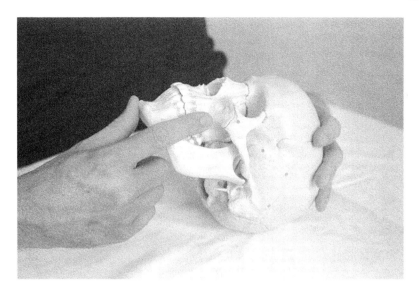

Movement	As for the mandible.
Comments	Tensions in the facial region can be trauma related – assault, falls, auto accident. As well as the obvious biomechanical forces that accompany the trauma, long-term loss of sensory acuity will occur. This is a highly significant zone for the internal mapping of the body. This loss of internal proprioceptive and sensory coherence can have catastrophic consequences in terms of loss of local postural controls. Over time this can lead to far-reaching consequences for the whole body.

LATERAL PTERYGOIDS

Client	As for above. Head rolled 10° to the ipsilateral side.
Therapist	Sitting on a stool at the shoulder level.
Technique	Use the little finger. Place it between the teeth and the coronoid process of the mandible (Figs 9.3, 9.4). (This is outside the teeth, not inside the mouth itself.) Direct the finger at the area of the TMJ by pointing it at the external auditory meatus. Ask the client to lateralize the jaw to the ipsilateral side to open up more space for the finger. Sink further toward the ear, without overpressure. Release may take anywhere between 45 and 120 seconds.
Movement	Although I love active client movement, this is one release where I'm inclined toward a more passive approach. Verbal coaching that guides the client to ease in the breathing will greatly assist the opening. Once again, the sensations of new space, lightening and reduced stiffness will need time to explore.
Comments	A typical response to this release is 'wow'. The changes in space, shape and movement will be that dramatic.

Figure 9.3
Finger placement for the lateral pterygoid release.

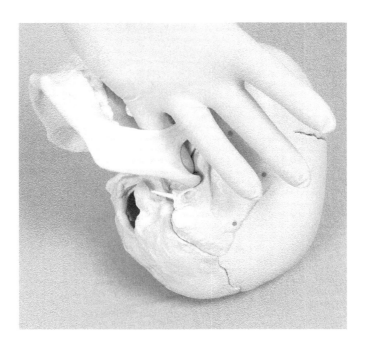

Figure 9.4
The left pterygoid muscles. The zygomatic arch and part of the ramus of the mandible have been removed (from Baldry PE 2001 Myofascial pain and fibromyalgia syndromes, with permission from Churchill Livingstone).

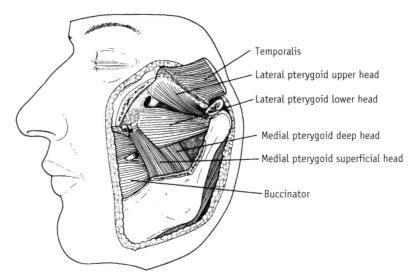

Temporalis

Lateral pterygoid upper head

Lateral pterygoid lower head

Medial pterygoid deep head

Medial pterygoid superficial head

Buccinator

MEDIAL PTERYGOID

Client

As for above.

Therapist

As for above.

Technique

The mouth is open. Use the first finger to contact the lateral aspect of the hard palate. Glide the finger along the palate in a posterior lateral direction until encountering the small raised bony bump at the beginning of the soft

Figure 9.5
Finger position for the inferior aspect of the medial pterygoid release.

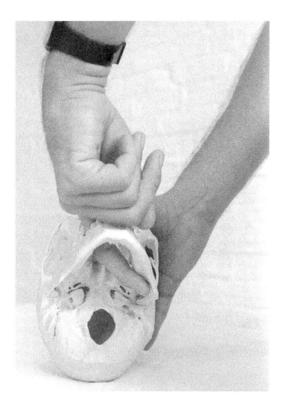

palate (Fig. 9.5). Glide over the bump and turn the movement toward the table (inferior). Avoid overpressure on the bony bump. The contact then moves from having a bony background to being solely on the soft tissue of the medial pterygoid. Maintain a steady pressure while moving toward the mandible. The contact can be carried onto the medial surface of the mandible.

Comments

The gag reflex will be activated by this contact in a few cases. Where direct contact with the muscle is prevented by gagging, simply work as close to the junction of the hard and soft palates as possible. The technique is modified by making it a 'hold and wait' type contact where firm pressure is maintained without any further posterior motion. Over 45–90 seconds there will be a general release through the whole zone.

Where the movement can be done without gag, be attentive to maintaining a melting intent rather than the unpleasant 'stripping' action that some therapies employ here.

FASCIAE OF THE HARD PALATE

Client

Supine with a small amount of capital extension.

Therapist

As for above.

Technique

Work on the ipsilateral side. Position the first finger as described above. This time the movement along the lateral aspect of the palate is more deliberate, with

Figure 9.6
Contacting the
anterior/lateral aspect
of the palate.

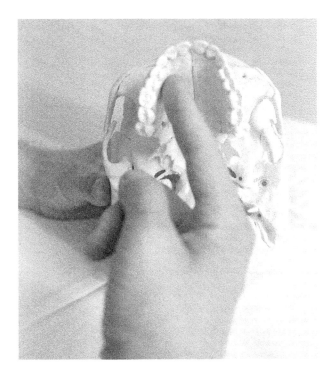

the introduction of a moderate amount of pressure. The tip as well as portions of the pad can be used for this. While traveling posteriorly and maintaining a lateral pressure, the forearm is pronated so that the finger rolls under the dome of the palate, producing a spreading effect, away from the midline (Fig. 9.6).

Comments

This feels fantastic when done well. The key to success is to keep a sense of saying hello to the soft tissue sensory fibers in the palatine fascia rather than a biomechanical intent. The movement is done slowly so that the client is able to 'find' the sensations and meet them. Once this feedback is established, all kinds of desirable changes in muscle tone, proprioceptive acuity and the ANS will take place. No need to force the issue at all!

PEDIATRIC SUPPLEMENT FOR THE INTRAORAL RELEASES

These intraoral releases are enormously useful for infants and children with a wide range of coordination and perceptual difficulties. They can augment existing therapies dealing with feeding, speech and head placement. While the initial model we developed to explain this effect was based on a change in the mechanical properties of fascia, it has become clear that it is the stimulation of the intrafascial sensory fibers that creates the beautiful changes in tone, control and coordination that we see. For example, stimulation of the muscle-free hard palate led to rapid changes in tone in the surrounding muscles, better head placement and control, improved tongue placement and so on.

While we too are highly suspicious of claims for the 'meta' usefulness of any one approach, we feel that these direct technique intraoral releases are excellent resources for physical, occupational and speech therapists.

Placing a child or infant in a supine position for intraoral work may be counterproductive. Various types of guarding may be aroused. Alternative positions can be explored. Infants and small children can be cradled (Fig. 9.7). Older children can be worked on sitting up or lying on their side (Figs 9.8, 9.9).

Figure 9.7
Cradling a child for intraoral MFR.

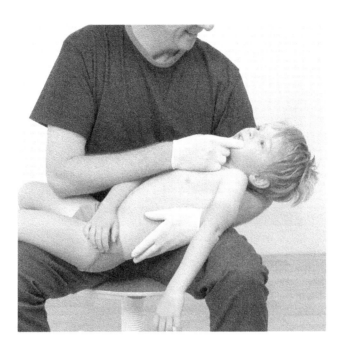

Figure 9.8
Working in sidelying position for intraoral work on a child.

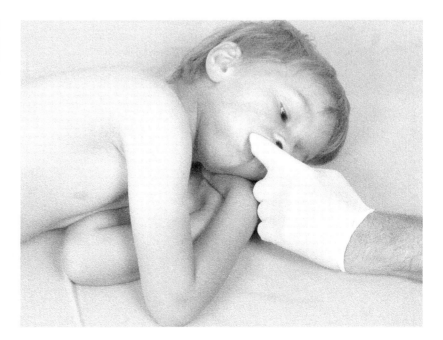

Figure 9.9
Doing intraoral work with
a child seated.

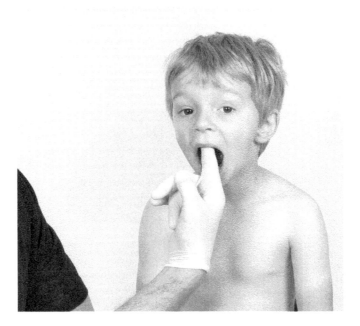

Chapter 10
THE CERVICAL REGION

LATERAL/ANTERIOR CERVICAL

Client Supine. Head slightly elevated if needed to prevent positional discomfort, with a folded towel, etc. No pillow.

Therapist Seated at the client's head. Shift the stool to the ipsilateral side so that the angle of contact is at around 45° to the client's neck.

Technique **1.** Rotate the head about 30° away from the side being treated. Make a soft fist and engage the mastoid process with the first phalange just distal to the MP joint (Fig. 10.1). Sink and engage firstly the thin layer of soft tissue and

Figure 10.1
Using a soft fist to treat the fascia at the mastoid process.

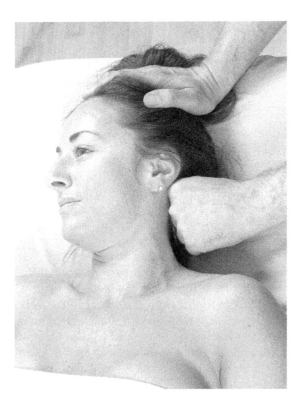

then the periosteum. Develop a line of tension and carry this posteriorly, around onto the occiput and as far into the midline of the head as possible.

2. Follow a similar protocol for the soft tissues that lie sub mastoid and occipital. With this contact it's possible to utilize a soft fist that uses the proximal portion of the first three phalanges. The effect of this will be not only to engage the periosteum of the bones but also broadly influence the deep and superficial layers of the superficial fascia of the anterior and lateral neck (Fig. 10.2).

Figure 10.2
Using the first three MP joints to treat the submastoid and occipital soft tissue.

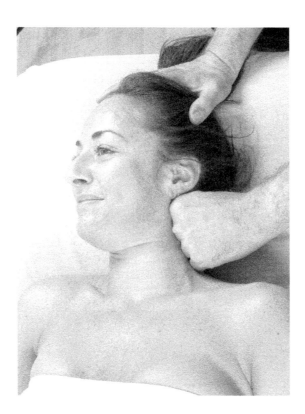

3. Treat the SCM, scalenes, levator scapula, splenius capitis and the superficial investing layer of the deep cervical fascia simultaneously. Use the pads of the index, middle and ring fingers to engage with the superior portion of the SCM, approximately 2 cm inferior to the mastoid process (Fig. 10.3). The index finger will be slightly anterior to that muscle's belly; the ring finger will be slightly posterior. Sink until a clear sense of contact with transverse processes of the cervical vertebrae can be felt. Take up a line of tension in an inferior direction. Keep this line of tension and add another, this time in a posterior direction. The effect of this is to work through the tissue in a spiral that can be carried around as far into the posterior aspect of the neck as possible. Repeat this spiralling sequence at a number of sites, each more inferior than the next.

4. Use a broad section of the pad of the index finger to work into the area of soft tissue just superior to the clavicle. Start medial to the AC joint and the fibers of the trapezius. Depress the finger inferiorly until the tissue is well engaged, without overpressure (Fig. 10.4). Keep this soft, broad and firm pressure while

Figure 10.3
Multiplanar approach to treating the SCM, scalenes, levator scapula and deep cervical fascia.

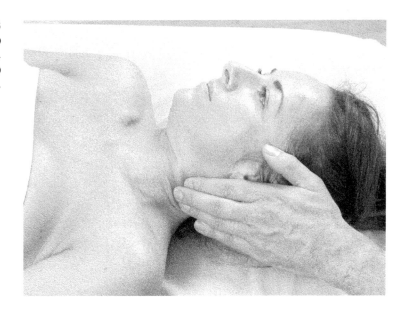

Figure 10.4
Releasing the fascia over the first rib.

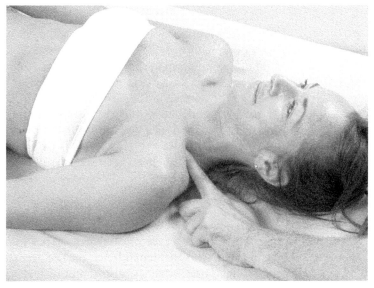

moving medially, towards the sternum. As the sternum is approached the first rib can often be felt releasing in the background. Continue the contact all the way to the clavicular tendon of the SCM.

5. Relocate the pad of the finger into the space between the clavicular and sternal portions of the SCM (Fig. 10.5). Apply a steady inferior pressure that deliberately seeks connection through to the first rib. This may take 30–45 seconds. You will feel the rib soften as it drops and the surrounding soft tissues will respond with increased pliancy and rapid reductions in stiffness.

Movement

Put the anterior flexor muscles off stretch by having the head adequately elevated without use of a pillow. Pillows produce too much fixed, non-dynamic flexion and impair the ability of these releases to facilitate fresh proprioceptive inputs.

Figure 10.5
Approaching the first rib via the space between the two portions of the SCM.

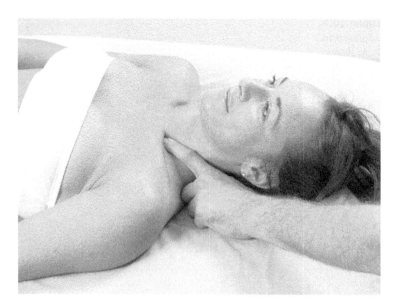

With their eyes open, have the client roll their head to the contralateral side. This is done without lifting the head off the table/towel. Encourage exploration of the sensation in the back of the head and side of the face sliding over the surface of the underlying material: 'Roll your head away from my contact and let your eyes take in the wall/picture/vase'. This roll to the contralateral side can be augmented with the suggestion to look over the shoulder on that same side. This induces a beautiful spiralling motion that serves to open out not only the front of the neck but also the whole anterior aspect of the upper trunk. Coach them to keep the eyes open and engaged with the room: 'Let your eyes take in the shadows/colors/shapes over your left/right shoulder'.

Comments   Whiplash is associated with microtrauma to all the soft tissues addressed in the preceding section. These releases will offer a lot of relief and resolution for that population. Overdependence on the accessory breathing muscles will produce SCMs and scalenes of steel and stiff, elevated first ribs. Chronic anxiety states that find their expression via the flexor muscles of the anterior hip, trunk and neck will generate a similar change in tissue texture and diminished proprioceptive acuity. While stabilizing approaches like Pilates are important in the long-term reeducation of these coordination problems, direct technique MFR is important to help restore mobility and, perhaps even more importantly, sensory awareness.

INFRAHYOID REGION

Client   As for above with slight capital extension and rotated 10–20° to the contralateral side.

Therapist   Seated on a stool at approximately mid-chest level or standing at the same level.

Technique

Use the pads of the first two fingers, or one only if your fingers are large, to take up a contact between the sternal portion of the SCM and the trachea, about 1–2 cm above the manubrium of the sternum (Fig. 10.6). Take up a superior line of tension and carry this up to the hyoid bone. This will affect the sternohyoid, omohyoid and sternothyroid muscles as well as the infrahyoid fascia and portions of the carotid sheath.

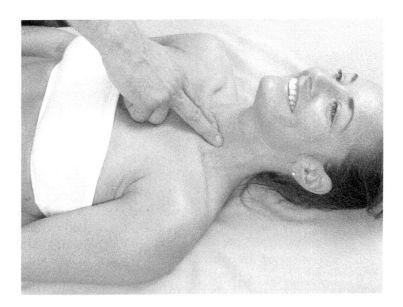

Figure 10.6
Release of the infrahyoid region.

Movement

Coach the client to slightly increase the length in the front of their neck: 'Roll your head back slightly to open this area under my fingers here'. This brings attention to movement as a lengthening, direction-oriented process rather than a blind, shortening one. Of course, this is important everywhere in the body but poorly coordinated movement and uncertain proprioception in the neck and head have really global implications for overall posture and balance.

Comments

This work must be done unilaterally. This is probably obvious but I thought I'd mention it just in case someone attempts to get creative and work bilaterally. It can be scary to have work done near some of the most important neurovascular structures in the body. Watch for muscle guarding, holding the breath and other defense mechanisms.

SUPRAHYOID REGION

Client

As for above.

Therapist

As for above.

Technique

Make contact with the pads of the first two fingers into the soft tissues immediately superior to the thyroid cartilage/hyoid bone (Fig. 10.7). Sink slightly to

Figure 10.7
Release of the suprahyoid
region.

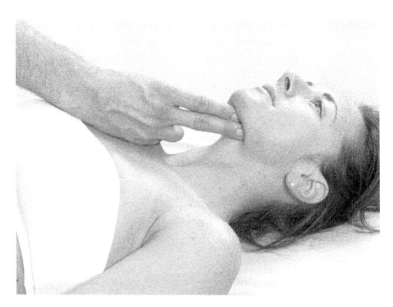

further engage the deep superficial fascia as well as the underlying muscular fasciae associated with the digastric. Develop a superior/lateral line of tension that works up into the floor of the mouth as well as across towards the angle of the mandible. Contact can be made with the periosteum of the medial aspect of the mandible.

Comments

This anterior zone of the neck is often ignored or undertreated in many soft tissue approaches to resolving whiplash. Experience shows that including all the anterior cervical myofasciae will more fully bring this condition to resolution.

An interesting component of restriction in this region is that it is often outside people's awareness. Tightness, pain and stiffness are reported in the posterior aspect yet palpatory and range-of-motion tests will frequently show that these anterior structures are involved in cervical restriction. Therefore it's useful to include an evaluation of these anterior structures with any cervical condition we might encounter.

There's an old saying, 'You don't have to feel bad to feel better'. This work, as well as the intraoral releases, has a lot to offer singers, actors and professional speakers. Finding ease and space throughout the head, neck, mouth and thorax gives new possibilities for vocal production and support. This can include the dissolution of existing patterns of tension associated with overexerting the voice. Stimulation of the intrafascial and intramuscular sensory fibers will give a spontaneous increase in proprioceptive awareness, which in turn will influence coordination. The nuances of support and voice placement will be immediately apparent once the sensory awareness has increased. This is good stuff for anyone who's already singing, acting or speaking and wants to improve without effort.

LONGUS COLLI

Client

As for above.

Therapist

As for above.

Technique

Use the pads of the first two fingers or one only if your fingers are large. Take up a contact between the sternal portion of the SCM and the trachea. Supinate the forearm slightly so that the pads of the fingers turn in to touch the trachea while the tips of the fingers are directed posteriorly (toward the table) (Fig. 10.8). This makes a more pointed contact than for the previous release of the superficial tissues. Keep the finger pads abutting the trachea and move gently to the contralateral side and open out a larger valley for the fingers to sink toward the anterior surface of the vertebrae. Take up a line of tension in a superior direction until there is a clear sense that to go any further would require overpressure and noxious sensation for the client.

Figure 10.8
Release of longus colli. Although this looks similar to the infrahyoid work the intention is to the very front of the cervical vertebrae. The bones can easily be felt during this release.

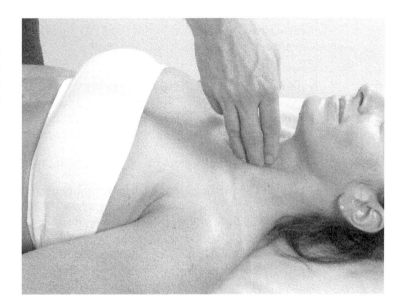

Movement

As for above. A variation can also be developed. Reach behind the neck with the other hand and place two or three fingers on the posterior surface of the vertebra, opposite to the site of contact on the anterior side. The lengthening process can now be guided with two points of specific sensory reference. Coach the client to make the opposite motion, this time taking the neck into a very local flexion motion. This isolation can be encouraged by asking the client to push back into the fingers that are lifting against the posterior aspect of the vertebra: 'Push just this one vertebra back into my fingers … right here'. This is done while there is deliberate counterpressure from those fingers to increase the sensory inputs and make the movement more likely.

Comments

In presenting direct technique MFR to massage therapists for over 15 years, I have observed an ongoing culture of fear around doing any specific work on the neck, especially the deeper myofasciae. The introduction into massage training of awareness of the vertebral artery and the possibility of occluding it during certain combinations of backward bending and rotation seems to have confirmed this fear. Add in the brachial plexus, facial nerve, carotid arteries and jugular veins and the region has become in the minds of many therapists a minefield that is best avoided. This is regrettable, as soft tissue approaches to the neck are so very important – the best approach in many instances – for a wide range of conditions.

Advocating the complete abandonment of caution would, of course, be reckless and irresponsible and all the protocols regarding medical assessment of acute injuries, referral and duty of care will always apply. The most obvious example of this is the need for X-ray after a whiplash injury to ascertain if there are fractures in the vertebrae. Deep work on an undiagnosed fracture could be catastrophic. I use this as an example because it is relatively likely that a client might present with a recent whiplash that has not been fully assessed.

Where direct technique MFR becomes the treatment of choice for many neck conditions is in the resolution of chronic stiffness. Yes, it's possible to exercise reasonable caution *and* do excellent, useful work in all the deeper cervical myofasciae, as described in this book. As always … slow, slow, slow.

Once again, do this work unilaterally!

DEEP POSTERIOR MYOFASCIAE

Client   Supine. Cervical spine at neutral. Positioned at least 10 cm away from the top of the table to allow room for the therapist's elbows and forearm to rest on the table.

Therapist   Seated on a stool at the head of a table, with the elbows supported on it.

Technique   Start at C7. Work bilaterally. The ring fingers are touching each other at the midline, over the spinous processes. Now lift the first three fingers of both hands broadly into the posterior aspect of the cervical spine (Fig. 10.9). This is best accomplished by supporting the elbows and forearms on the table. Then deliberately push them both further into the table which will lift the fingers anteriorly and more firmly against the vertebrae. The head is cradled in the fore-arms. Maintain the anterior pressure and introduce a superior line of tension. The ring and middle fingers are able to go directly onto the nuchal ligament during this. The head is rotated into chin tuck position as the arms are pulled

Figure 10.9
Release of the nuchal ligament. The fingertips are lifting into the spinous processes.

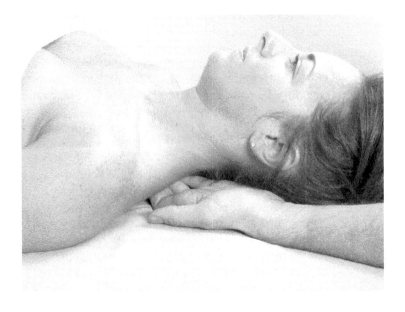

superiorly. The firm anterior pressure is maintained while the line of tension extends to the suboccipital triangle.

Work bilaterally. Reach under the posterior portion of the lower cervical spine and lift the tips of the first two fingers of each hand into the lamina grooves at the level of C7–T1 (Fig. 10.10). This is best accomplished by supporting the elbows and forearms as described earlier. Increase the anterior pressure and then add a lateral line of tension. This brings a slow melting effect to the myofasciae behind the transverse processes. Repeat this process of deliberate lifting, spreading and melting at each vertebra up to C2.

Figure 10.10
Melting into the deep, small muscles of the posterior neck.

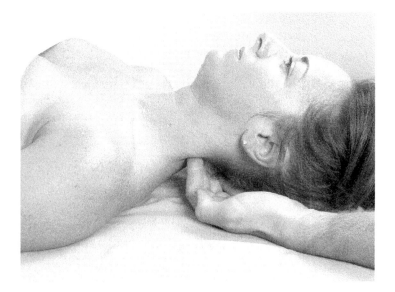

Work bilaterally. Position the fingers as for release number 2. This time maintain a static anterior pressure. Coach the client to push this single vertebra further back into your fingers (Fig. 10.11). The focus is on each individual segment. Work each spinal segment up to C2.

Figure 10.11
Activating the deep flexor muscles via precise segmental pressure with coordinated movement.

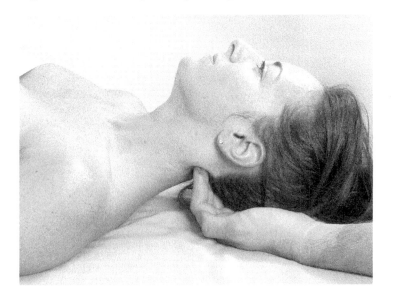

Movement

Direct the client to put both arms, with palms down, onto the table. While the neck is lengthened by you, the therapist, ask them to slide their hands along the table, toward their feet. At the same time encourage them to allow the upper back to feel wide – encouraging the breath to the sides of the body can assist with this: 'Lift your fingers slightly and open your palms into the table ... now slide your palms across the table towards your feet'.

Ask for slight, non-specific (wriggling, twisting, pulsing) micro movements that connect to the segment being touched.

Coach the client towards the use of the intrinsic muscles and away from the use of the big neck flexors. Monitor the scalenes and SCM; point out when they fire and encourage patient exploration of a new movement. The strong contact into the vertebra will give lots of sensory input to assist with this isolation of intrinsic motion.

Comments

The third release works to reactivate muscles that have been rendered mute by the loud thunder of the big muscles. It's a delightful way to quickly integrate the function of the neck after the preceding deep releases. I recommend always finishing with this.

RELEASE OF THE CRANIAL BASE AND THE SUBOCCIPITAL MYOFASCIAE

Client

Supine. Positioned to allow the therapist's forearms to rest on the table.

Therapist

Seated on a stool at the head of the table. Elbows and supinated forearms on the table.

Technique

Ask the client to lift their head off the table. Position the tips of the first three fingers into the soft tissue immediately inferior to the occiput (Fig. 10.12).

Figure 10.12
Release of the suboccipital region, including the triangle.

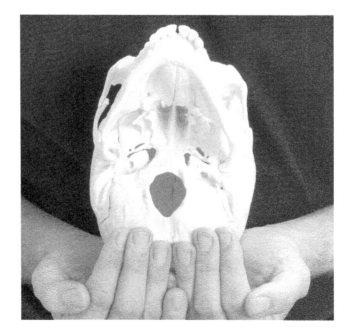

The two index fingers are abutting each other at the midline. The fingers are stabilized in a flexed position – around 45° at the MP and PIP joints. The client is asked to rest their head back down so the fingertips are in the suboccipital soft tissues and the fingerpads rest firmly against the inferior aspect of the occiput. The head is also supported by the thenar eminences, at about the level of the superior nuchal line of the occiput.

Once the position is perceived to be comfortable, a series of soft tissue responses will occur, characterized by local softening sensations followed by an increase in the weight of the head. (There is no superior traction during this phase.) Next, develop a line of tension through the suboccipital tissues, as well as into the periosteum of the occiput, by separating the two hands. This is done by supinating the forearms which will lead to the two hands being pulled apart from each other.

Another cycle of release will commence, with associated changes in local tissue texture and tonus as well as broad regional changes via the effects on the ANS. Once this cycle is well established, experiment with the addition of slight superior traction – perhaps 20–30 grams of effort. If there is strong tissue recoil, then moderate the force.

Movement

Try offering an image to augment the softening and widening effect: 'Let the back of your head grow wide'. Another useful one to offer is the possibility that the 'eyes can soften and rest back into the head'.

Comments

A smooth uptake of the release, that does not require the client to lift their head, can be mastered. Roll the head to one side and slide the contralateral hand into its position as described above. Now use the ipsilateral hand to roll the head up onto the fingers and thenar eminence of the newly positioned hand. Lift the head sufficiently with that hand to allow the other hand to take up its position next to it. Return the head back to the midline. The hands are symmetrically placed. Now further engage the fingers into the suboccipital traingle by 'scooping' the hands along the table in an inferior direction while simultaneously lifting the fingers anteriorly. The head should rotate about an axis drawn between the ears. Now the suboccipital triangle is contacted at the fingertips and the thenar eminences will be able to support that by stabilizing at the mastoid process. Once mastered, this takes just a few seconds.

Hypertonicity of the muscles of the suboccipital triangle is a central component of tension headaches. Mastering this approach to these intrinsic soft tissues will be of enormous benefit in effectively treating this condition. Combine it with MFR to the larger muscles of the region: trapezius, splenius capitis and cervicis, longissimus capitus, semispinalis capitis. These larger muscles have considerable mechanical advantage on the occiput and unloading them prior to releasing the suboccipital triangle is a recommended strategy. For more information on treating tension headaches, see Chapter 12.

A common outcome with a deep release of the suboccipital muscles is a shift in ANS tonus throughout the entire body. This is initially most apparent in the changes to respiration as the frequency is generally lowered. The accessory breathing muscles, tied to the SNS, relax as the PNS activity increases. Spontaneous belly breathing, with a prolonged preinspiration phase, occurs. There will often be an involuntary shift into a hypnogogic state with an associated increase in muscular twitching and jerking. While the client is drifting in this state between awake and asleep, dream-like images may appear. If time allows, this can be a wonderful state to let the client float along in. It's profoundly relaxing and often is the body seeking a reorientation toward the PNS with its powerful restorative and regenerative functions. Other signs of this shift toward the PNS include borborygmus (bowel sounds – gurgling and the like), drooling and, less frequently, an extremely rapid opening and closing of the jaw (like shivering) with the teeth clicking on each other.

DECOMPRESSION OF THE OCCIPITAL CONDYLES

Client   As above.

Therapist   As above.

Technique   Make a stand out of the first and middle fingers (as shown in Fig. 10.13). The middle fingers of each hand abut each other. For easiest application of the technique, simply ask the client to lift their head to allow your prepositioned hands

Figure 10.13
Further release of the suboccipital triangle region.

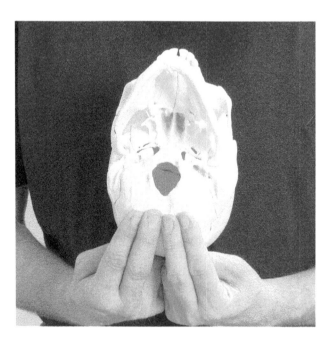

into place. As the client rests back onto your fingers, hook under the occiput so that the fingertips are pointing anterior/superior. The mastoid processes are resting on the thenar eminences (not shown in the photo) and the thumbs can assist with stability. Introduce superior traction. This is very light and without any semblance of overpressure – perhaps 10–15 grams of effort. Now add a similar traction in a posterior direction, towards the table. The occipital base will progressively relax away from the top of the neck. As the space here opens, reposition the fingertips so that they are even more 'under' the occiput. Continue the intent to translate the occiput into the table or into the floor.

| Movement | Ask for an exaggerated inhale and coach the client to hold their breath momentarily before allowing the exhale out through their mouth with a relaxed jaw. This is not a forced exhalation but more like a big sigh. Point out that this is not a recommended breathing pattern to take further into the session, or beyond it. |

| Comments | This technique is presented as the release of bony articulations, the condyles, yet I find the work proceeds better when I do not think so much in terms of biomechanics. I like to keep my intention at the level of the sustained stimulation of the fasciae and periosteum; in other words, the intrafascial mechanoreceptors. This is communication – a long hello to the local residents of the suboccipital regions. |

PEDIATRIC SUPPLEMENT FOR THE CERVICAL REGION

Modification of the client position will be necessary for many of these releases. Receiving work in the supine position will not always be possible. The releases that follow are designed to approach the same regions covered in the preceding section from different perspectives.

LATERAL/ANTERIOR MYOFASCIAE IN SIDELYING

| Client | Sidelying position. |

| Therapist | Generally, work from behind. Working from in front is possible although getting the angles of contact can be more challenging. |

| Technique | Make a soft fist. Contact the anterior portion of the mastoid process with the proximal portion of the first phalange (Fig. 10.14). Take up a line of tension in a posterior direction. Carry this line across onto the occiput and as far towards the midline as possible. This can also be done with the pad of a finger(s). |

Figure 10.14
Sidelying approach to releasing the soft tissue of the temporal bone and occiput.

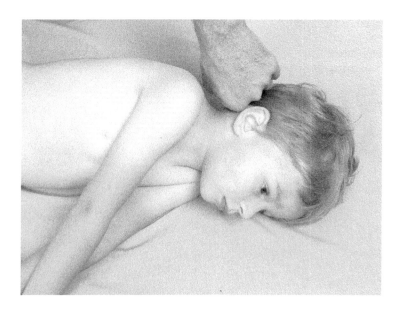

Use a soft fist. Position the first MP or PIP joint sub mastoid and allow the other MP or PIP joints, and the proximal portions of the phalanges if using the MPs, to sink slightly and broadly engage the soft tissues of the lateral neck (Fig. 10.15). Develop a line of tension by following the contours of the neck around toward the nuchal ligament. This can also be done with the pad of a finger(s).

Figure 10.15
Sidelying approach to releasing the SCM, scalenes and deep cervical fascia.

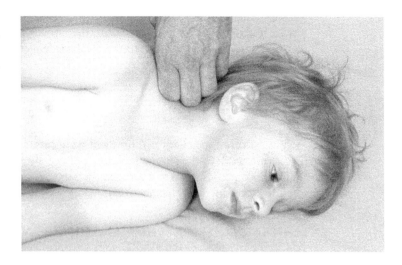

Position yourself superior to and slightly behind the child. Use the finger-pad of the first two fingers to engage the space just superior of the clavicle, immediately medial to the fibers of the trapezius (Fig. 10.16). The other hand can be used to elevate and internally rotate the shoulder until the tissues under the pad of the finger go slack. This enables a fuller engagement into the fascia along the superior surface of the first rib. Develop a line of tension toward the sternum. Maintain some degree of inferior pressure throughout.

Figure 10.16
Release of the first rib and associated soft tissue in sidelying.

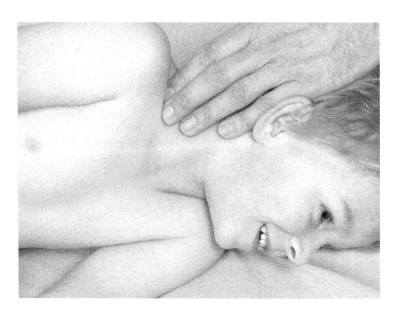

Reposition so that you are now behind and at the level of the shoulder. Face superiorly. Use the lower hand to once again elevate the shoulder so that the trapezius is put on slack. Use the tip/pad of the first two fingers to engage the lateral tissue of the neck just anterior to the fibers of the trapezius (Fig. 10.17). This will be slightly posterior to the transverse process of C6. Maintain the engagement, at the level of the periosteum if possible, and develop a line of tension toward the mastoid process.

Figure 10.17
Release of the deeper, small neck muscles in sidelying position.

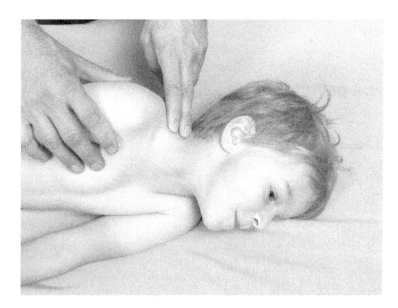

Movement

While one hand is saying hello to the myofasciae of the lateral head and neck, the other hand can introduce a lovely rotation to the contralateral side (into the pillow/table). Use the broad surface of the hand for this to give lots of sensation – warmth and pressure – around the face while the movement is being facilitated. Add a nodding motion as well and there will be a smooth spiral of movement for the child to orient their proprioception around.

Chapter 11
THE HEAD AND FACE

According to the body's internal map of itself, the head, especially the face and mouth, is the center of the bodily universe; 38% of the neurologic input to the brain comes from the face, mouth and TMJ region. To talk about affecting the person via individual muscles in this region is especially spurious. The body map relates to it as a sea of sensation, not as bits and pieces. Still, with that caveat in mind, muscles will be included in these descriptions as a navigational convenience rather than with any thought that 'treating' them as individuals is possible, or desirable for that matter.

MASSETER

Client   Supine.

Therapist   Seated at the head of the table.

Technique   Work bilaterally. Use the pads of the first three fingers to engage the soft tissue over the zygomatic arch. The ring finger is on the zygomatic process of the temporal bone, approximately 1 cm anterior to the ear (Fig. 11.1). The middle

Figure 11.1
MFR for the superficial and deep portions of the masseter.

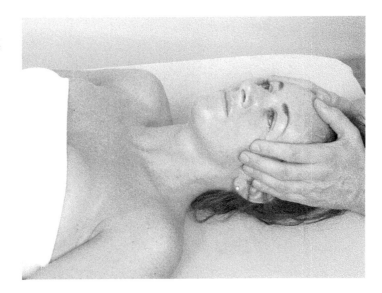

finger is contacting the mid-portion of that process; the first finger is contacting the temporal process of the zygomatic bone. Sink through the soft tissue until the bone is clearly contacted. Maintain this connection with the periosteum and introduce an inferior line of tension, towards the angle of the mandible. Twist the fingers slightly to increase the local shearing effect in the fascia. Carry this line of tension onto the mandible, where the periosteum is also engaged. Repeat a number of times. Deepen the intention from the superficial masseter to its deeper portion.

Movement

Ask for micro movements of the jaw; wiggling, spiraling motions will be more useful than simply asking for the mouth to open and close.

Comments

When the mandible is engaged, an inferior tractioning action can be introduced. The focus of this is not on stretching per se but a sustained pressure into the periosteum, delivered with a sense of direction. This will quite quickly lead to a change in local tonus as well as sensations of release on a more regional scale as well. The suboccipital zone can open, tensions in the breathing and the deep constrictors in the throat can relax.

ZYGOMATICUS MAJOR AND MINOR

Client

Supine.

Therapist

Seated at the head of the table.

Technique

Work bilaterally. Use the pads of the first two fingers. Engage the inferior surface of the zygomatic arch approximately 2 cm anterior to the ear (Fig. 11.2). The contact is deliberately against the periosteum. Develop a line of tension and carry this anterior, tracing the zygomatic arch to the zygomatic bones, then onto the maxillae.

Figure 11.2
MFR for the major and minor zygomatic muscles.

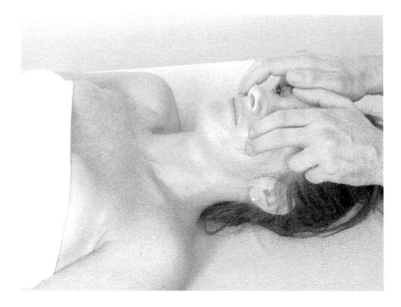

| **Movement** | As for above. |

| **Comments** | This can be repeated a number of times. The intention is on stimulation of sensation. Avoid overpressure of the kind that might accompany a well-intended attempt to stretch tight muscles. |

TEMPORALIS FASCIA

| **Client** | Sidelying, head supported at neutral by a pillow. |

| **Therapist** | Standing behind client at the level of the shoulders, facing superiorly. |

| **Technique** | Use the pads of the first 2–3 fingers of each hand to engage the soft tissues immediately above the ear (Fig. 11.3). The contact will fan around the ear – the most anterior finger will be on the anterior portions of the temporal process of the zygomatic bone, the most posterior on the posterior section of the parietal bone, depending on the head/hand size ratio. Sink firmly. The head will be pushed deeply into the pillow/folded towel. Maintain this deliberate pressure and then put in a very local line of superior tension – a micro stretch. Continue with a series of these engagements – sink, add a local line of tension, wait, release, reposition, repeat. Avoid 'raking' through the hair. Work in increments up to the epicranial aponeurosis and carry the work as close to the top of the head as possible. |

Figure 11.3
MFR to the temporalis muscle.

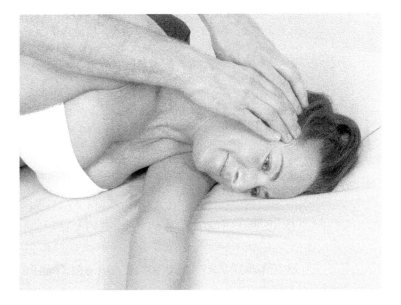

| **Movement** | Micro movements of the jaw (wiggling/yawning) and head (nodding/wobbling) will augment the opening and release in this region. |

| **Comments** | Curiously, the work in the hair is rarely painful. In fact, the opposite is true – most people go into a deep PNS state during this work. This is terrific stuff for general stress reduction. It is also indicated for a wide range of head and TMJ |

problems, especially headaches with a strong clenched jaw component. There will often be multiple tender points in the muscle and its tendon. These warrant special attention. My recommendation, though, is to blend these local releases into the surrounding tissue as this is more beneficial than excessive local intent.

Cranial sacral therapies, whatever their origin or trademark protected name, all make various claims about affecting the deepest membranes and fluids of the body, as well as the bones within the cranium, spine and sacrum. Explanations of the work range from the mechanical to the neurologic and even to the flat-out esoteric.

The efficacy of these various approaches can be augmented by thoroughly addressing the soft tissues around the cranium and face. Freeing the strain that is so common in these various myofasciae will make for easier entry into the more subtle levels of the so-called cranial sacral system. It is certainly my consistent observation that we can move seamlessly into the dreamy, tidal world of lightest touch cranial work from direct technique MFR done in any of the myofasciae of the body. However, this ability is especially potent when doing MFR around the head and face.

Clearly, research and observation tell us that direct technique MFR favorably influences the ANS. Equally as obvious, although there is an absence of research to confirm it, is the fact that cranial sacral therapy is engaging the ANS as well. While the cranial approach generally draws from the lightest end of the spectrum of touch and direct technique MFR somewhat from the middle, they elicit a number of common responses.

Hugh Milne DO has written the beautifully titled *The Heart of Listening* which encapsulates in a single phrase the essence of his approach to cranial sacral therapy. Still, when we analyze any touch therapy, from the most subtle to the firmest, they all have a strong 'hello' component as well. Perhaps the order is 'hello' then we 'listen' for the response, respond to that with an 'ah' or a 'hmmm' or a 'there', send a new 'hello', 'listen' to see how it is taken, and so on. This is the essence of communication as relationship, a view that moves away from the transmission model (I send the signal that you will receive just as I intended) to a more open-ended one (let's see what happens now we've engaged in this way). This dynamic can develop with contact from a number of points along the spectrum of touch, not just the lightest.

I recommend that the next time a cranial session appears not to be having an effect – no hynogogia, relaxation, twitching, tidal waves, etc. – shift the focus to the myofasciae around the face. Think of it as a fresh 'hello' and see if there is a shift in what you are 'listening' to soon after. Develop the art of saying 'hello' in a variety of ways by drawing on a broader lexicon of touch.

EPICRANIAL APONEUROSIS (OR GALEA APONEUROTICA)

Client

Supine.

Therapist

Seated on a stool at the head of the table. Shift the stool to angle on to the head at 45°.

Technique

Stabilize the head with one hand via light touch on the forehead. Use the pads of the fingers of the other hand to work through the hair, if there is some, and engage the fibrous tissue over the bones (Fig. 11.4). Take the contact against the bone, without overpressure, and develop small, local lines of tension, as for the temporalis fascia. Continue with a systematic treatment of the whole region until tissue pliancy is clearly improved.

Figure 11.4
MFR to the epicranial aponeurosis.

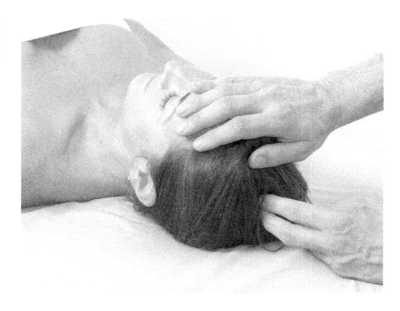

Movement	Any general movement of the facial muscles will add a useful counterpressure.
Comments	Tension here and in the muscles that use the aponeurosis as a central tendon is common. This tension is often underappreciated and thus ignored in approaches to working with headaches. Releasing it feels delightful. Observe rapid reductions in SNS activity with associated full-body reductions in tonus.

PROCERUS AND NASALIS MUSCLES

Client	Supine.
Therapist	Seated on a stool at the head of the table.
Technique	One hand is placed across the frontal bone. The whole hand is making contact – heel, palm and fingers – so the pressure feels broad and comfortable. There is sufficient weight applied to feel through the soft tissues onto the periosteum. Now position the other hand so that it can rest on the one placed over the frontal bone, with the first finger and thumb lightly 'pinching' the nose (Fig. 11.5). The contact should be broadly through the pads as far lateral as the level of the orbits of the eyes. Develop a line of tension toward the distal nose while the hand on the frontal bone tethers the tissue in counterpoint. Take the contact all the way to the end of the nose. The pinching is only sufficient to engage the tissues; there is no squeezing.
Movement	Non-specific movements often work best. Smiling is good for the facial muscles.

Figure 11.5
MFR to the procerus and nasalis muscles.

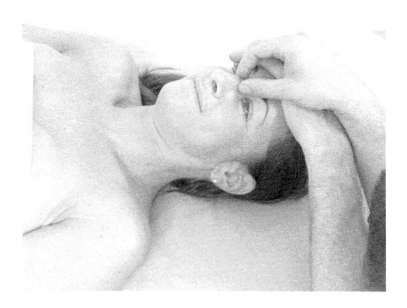

Comments   This can assist in clearing the frontal and maxillary sinuses.

POSTERIOR CRANIUM

Client   Supine.

Therapist   Seated on a stool at the head of the table.

Technique   Work with both hands and engage bilaterally. Cradle the head in the palms. The fingertips of the first three fingers can now lift into the posterior aspect of the cranium (Fig. 11.6). The initial contact is into the soft tissues at the

Figure 11.6
Position and direction for MFR to the myofasciae of the posterior cranium. Start at the inferior nuchal ridge, proceed to the superior nuchal ridge and beyond.

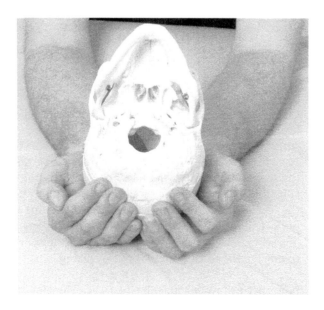

superior nuchal line of the occiput. Lift, engage and then establish a superior line of tension. Each line of tension is slight, just like the temporalis. Reposition and repeat in increments across the occiput and onto the parietal bones. Focus into the discrete zones of tenderness, puffiness and tension. Blend these local releases into the broader work across the whole region.

PEDIATRIC SUPPLEMENT FOR THE HEAD

While direct technique MFR produces consistent outcomes on the adult head, the same consistency has not been observed when working with CP children. The underlying dynamic for this is not clear. Coherent experimentation with a keen eye for the result is the best advice. Intraoral work is quite different and the huge benefits associated with this are elaborated on in Chapter 9.

TEMPORALIS FASCIA

Client Supine or in sidelying as per the previous release.

Therapist Position will vary depending on the surface.

Technique Work bilaterally. Make a contact above the ears with the pads of the first two fingers (Fig. 11.7). Establish superior lines of tension. Lightly rotate the tissues

Figure 11.7
Bilateral MFR to the
temporalis myofascia.

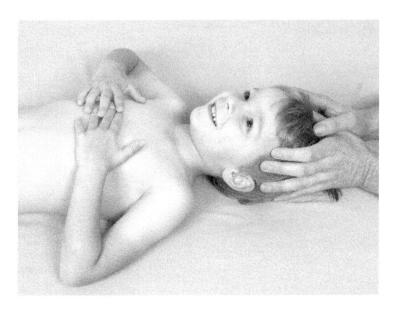

to the right and then the left. Ascertain if there is a barrier to one side or the other, i.e. the tissue will not rotate as far to one side as the other. Work lightly against the barrier. Coax the tissue to go against this bind. This is not forceful but feels like twisting a cork to move it out of the neck of a bottle. It adds another plane of fascial tension. Work in increments, with attention to the long spirals of multiplanar tensions.

Comments   Part of the experimentation will be to ascertain where on the spectrum of touch to work. Try various pressures and observe the response. Look for signs of PNS activation to confirm the usefulness of a depth. If it's not forthcoming after 30 seconds or so, shift to another level.

Chapter 12

TOWARDS THE MORE EFFECTIVE TREATMENT OF HEADACHES

Almost all endogenous headaches are characterized by multiple areas of tenderness and hypertonicity in the area of the occiput and the suboccipital region. This includes the suboccipital triangle but is not confined to it. These areas generally remain tender even during periods when the person is without a headache. They may be primary or secondary features of the headache syndrome. Treatment of these soft tissue restrictions and congestions is generally successful using the methodology outlined in this book. Since headaches are so commonly reported in client histories, presenting a comprehensive approach to treating them will be useful.

For the purposes of this chapter, conditions such as hypertonicity, soft tissue contractures, myofascial restriction and trigger point formation are seen to involve interrelated physiologic, neurologic, psychologic and psychosocial processes in a dynamic feedback loop. This kind of interrelationship approach was elaborated upon in the Introduction. To review briefly, this more inclusive view enables the functional anatomy of the cranium, cervical and thoracic spines and the pelvic floor to be seen as a complex of interdependent structures and processes. The significance of the ANS in providing the body with its self-regulatory function is also restated.

THERAPEUTIC GOALS

The cranial base

The initial goal of therapy for a headache syndrome is to reduce the generalized hypertonicity of the suboccipital and occipital regions. Commence with broad MFR to the mastoid process of the temporal bone and extend this onto the occiput (see Chapter 10). Deep and superficial layers of myofasciae meet along bony landmarks. Work here has a desirable dispersive effect into the surrounding region. After this attention to broad release, treatment of localized tender points along the occiput can be commenced.

Search and treat bilaterally on the occiput (see Chapter 11, p150). Myofasciae from the cervical and thoracic spines have attachments in this zone. The larger ones, especially the trapezius, exert a considerable leverage on the cranial base. These releases should precede attention to the underlying suboccipital triangle.

After treatment of these discrete restrictions in the posterior cranium, blend the work back into the broader fasciae of the epicranial aponeurosis. Treat this region until movement and pliancy are restored. Fingers, knuckles and even the well-directed elbow can make this area come alive. If palpating for mobility here brings on a pleasure response – big sigh, reductions in tonus or even a rapid hypnogogic state – but there are no obvious restrictions or tender points, carry on working to deepen the PNS response. Things don't have to feel bad to feel better!

Now release the suboccipital triangle by applying the two specific releases from Chapter 10 (pp138, 140). This stage of release will take several minutes. It involves a number of 'hellos' and 'listenings' as the response develops. This is one of the highest leverage sites in the body and the amount of change that comes from these releases can be truly impressive.

Thoracic outlet

Most emphasis in soft tissue therapies is given to the longitudinal muscles of the body. Rightly so, as they constitute the majority of tissue directly accessible to the therapist. However, the horizontal structures – the thoracic outlet, respiratory, pelvic and urogenital diaphragms and possibly the tentorium cerebellum – are potential barriers to the uninterrupted exchange of fluids (lymph, axoplasm, arterial and venous blood, etc.) throughout the body. Of course, these structures have received increased focus in recent times due to the attention given to them in cranial sacral therapy. The respiratory and pelvic diaphragms are now receiving more attention as their role in core stability is understood.

The thoracic outlet is a posited diaphragm. It is not a single muscle, nor a series of related ones like the pelvic floor. An inclusive definition combines the bones, muscles and fascia of the region. Tensions in the myofasciae are involved in the disruption of the flows needed to nourish the intra- and extracranial tissues.

Restriction in the thoracic outlet may cause congestion of the intra- and extracranial fluids in a fashion similar to chronic or acute suboccipital restrictions. The carotid artery, jugular vein, brachial plexus and vagus nerve all pass through this outlet. Restrictions to these deep neurovascular structures, as well as the many more superficial ones, is a common cause of headache, cranial malaise (non-specific feelings of disorientation, pressure and stiffness, often with fatigue), cervical pain and a component in peripheral neuropathies in the upper extremity.

Treatment begins with the MFR to the upper fibers of the trapezius. This can be done with the patient in the seated position (see Chapter 8, p92) or in prone. It's a common observation that prone position, with or without a face cradle, can exacerbate a headache in progress. The mechanism for this is unclear. Perhaps the pressure on the facial bones leads to an increase in pressure in the sinuses.

Next, work with the patient in supine position and treat the scalenes and other anterior lateral myofascia (see Chapter 10, p129). Next, give attention to releasing the first rib and its related fascia. Work patiently until the rib is clearly floating free (see Chapter 10, p131). This is not traditional mobilizing but an approach to releasing the rib in relationship to the surrounding soft tissues.

Attend to restrictions in the pectoralis major (see Chapter 8, p109) and minor. Use of one or more of the functional breathing releases may be necessary to fully release the overutilization of the pectorals, scalenes and SCM for breathing (see Chapter 8, p114).

ANS responses are common as release occurs. These include localized and whole-body twitching, eye fluttering and rapid changes in respiratory rhythm and amplitude. As with any ANS activity, it should be allowed, encouraged and followed to completion. This is the body's self-regulation at work and it should be supported. Verbal coaching to allow the responses rather than contain them may be helpful if there is fear around such strong involuntary motions. Since it is well established that people decompress and unravel in situations that are safe, reassurance that these are the normal releases of accumulated stress may be necessary. However, most clients have no doubt that this is the case as the release feels organic and satisfying.

Pelvic floor

A hypertonic pelvic floor will often cause compression of the distal portions of the vagus nerve and result in a range of visceral problems including digestive distress, bloating and cramping. These conditions are often present in the endogenous headache syndrome and treatment of this diaphragm can be part of their management.

Apply the pelvic traction described on p85. As well as assisting the pelvic floor to release, especially the chronically tight posterior portion, this will deepen the rebalancing occurring in the ANS. Other pelvic floor approaches can be helpful (see Chapter 7, p79).

TMJ and intraoral tensions

A more complete release of the cranial base can be accomplished via attention to the intraoral structures. Ask about bruxism, jaw pain, teeth that are painful/tender upon waking, clenching during the day or upon waking. Tensions in the suboccipital region can be exacerbated or caused through chronic tightness in the masseter (see Chapter 11, p145), pterygoids (see Chapter 9, pp124, 125) and temporalis muscles.

SELF-HELP

Several treatments will be necessary for the headaches to be resolved, diminished in frequency and/or severity. Providing patients with self-help techniques can be an important way to support the changes made through therapy as well as at its conclusion.

Teach clients how to treat the tender points along the superior nuchal ridge and in the suboccipital region. This can be done lying supine, sitting up or slumped over a desk to facilitate a reduction in the tone of the cervical muscles. Most people who suffer from recurrent tension headaches get good at knowing when one is possible or definitely on the way. Attention to diffusing the intensity of the neurophysiologic shifts that accompany the headache's onset can be done during periods of high emotional or environmental stress as a preventive measure.

Another useful method for easing these accumulating tensions is via resting the head on two tennis balls that have been tied together in a sock or stocking. The balls are held firmly next to each other by knotting the sock or stocking. The client lies supine with the tennis balls under the nuchal ridge of the occiput. This is, of course, somewhat like the position for the CV4 procedure in cranial sacral therapy. Many people find this relaxing; some will not, so experimentation is needed.

Recommend periods of rest throughout the day when the patient lies down and rests the cervical spine. The addition of a rolled-up towel under the cervicals can increase the relaxation. Some people respond well to sleeping on a specially contoured pillow. Once again, experiment.

Analgesics can be an important part of a person's response to the onset of a headache, particularly at times when more involved corrective exercises, autogenic relaxation approaches and the like are not possible. During travel, for example, it can be impossible to do much about the onset of a headache except take some form of medication to stop the development of a full-blown pain spasm, SNS arousal cycle. A well-known cranial teacher, whom I will not name, who suffered a very serious whiplash that impaired her ability to work for a number of years, told a class that when flying she sometimes got a headache. When asked what she did for the headache (I think the class expected an esoteric answer involving the breath of life and other intangibles), the answer was 'take aspirin'. This certainly left a lot of people flabbergasted. I thought it was refreshing. Clearly, there are numerous useful resources that can be employed as needed. However, as is well known, analgesics have toxic side-effects and do not offer any long-term solution to headaches.

Headaches may be a symptom of a more profound problem such as clinical depression, a tumor, vision problems, chronic sinus infection or severe allergies. The approaches to working with headaches outlined in this brief chapter are designed to expand the response ability of the soft tissue therapist, not to replace comprehensive and specialized diagnosis performed by a physician. When headaches are recurrent and/or severe, referral is always indicated.

Chapter 13
THE UPPER EXTREMITIES

CORACOID PROCESS

Client

Supine with the shoulder externally rotated, with the dorsum of the hand resting on the table next to the head. Arm abducted to 15°.

Therapist

Work from the contralateral side, especially if the client is large and your arms are short in relation to that. Otherwise working from the ipsilateral side is also acceptable.

Technique

The initial component of this release is described in the anterior trunk work in Chapter 8, p109. Extend this work onto the coracoid process and maintain the lateral/superior line of tension while resting on the bone. Slow it down. Now have the client take their arm into abduction while tethering the tissues over the bone (tendons of coracobrachialis, short head biceps brachii and pectoralis minor) (Fig. 13.1).

Figure 13.1
Using contact at the coracoid process to influence multiple tendons, myofasciae and periosteum.

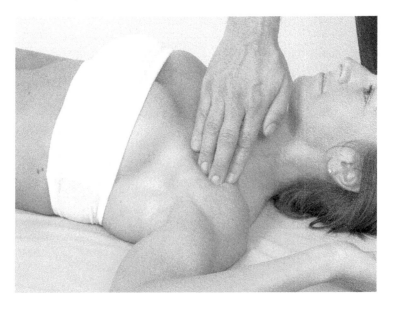

Movement

This can be micro movement if a large range of motion is uncomfortable. Try a few degrees of abduction and adduction. Narrow the range of oscillation until the movement is across just a centimeter or so. This starts to feel like an internal massage that is meeting the pressure to create increased release.

Comments

Just as restrictions in the anterior trunk have a strong occupational component, so too do the shoulder girdle and upper extremities. Ironically perhaps, manual therapists are especially vulnerable to postural instability, stiffness, diminished ROM and pain within the shoulder joints, wrists and smaller joints of the fingers. Almost all manual therapies require long periods of internal rotation of the shoulder with no counterbalancing external rotation. Scapula instability is also a problem. Most therapists will benefit from the application of these shoulder releases on themselves!

PECTORALIS MINOR

Client

Supine. The shoulder of the treated arm is internally rotated to the extent needed to have the palm of the hand resting on the stomach and the elbow on the table.

Therapist

Standing at the client's side, at the mid-thoracic level.

Technique

The therapist's forearm is pronated, i.e. palm is facing the floor. Use the tips/pads of the first three fingers to contact the rib cage immediately inferior to the lateral fibers of pectoralis major. This is the most anterior aspect of the axilla. Sink medially and contact both the soft tissues and the periosteum of the ribs. Make the contact as broad as possible. Now direct the fingertips at the client's chin, working under the pectoralis major. The fingers should extend into the pocket that lies between the pectoralis major and the ribs, with the pads contacting the ribs (Fig. 13.2). The tips will work against the lateral margin of the pectoralis minor.

Figure 13.2
Access to the pectoralis minor and upper ribs via the axilla.

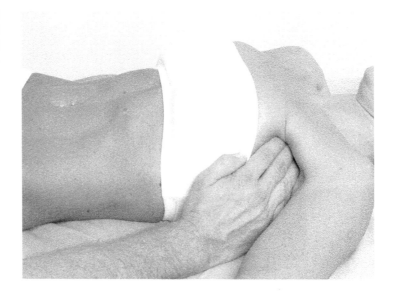

Movement

I used to teach this with the arm in abduction and external rotation. For many people this puts the tissue on too much stretch, causing the deep contact to be unnecessarily painful. If the work is well tolerated then have the client explore one or both of these motions. If guarding is the only response, desist. All clients will benefit from directing their attention to the tensions in the upper ribs and how the steady pressure can help release them. This attention can be encouraged through the breath: 'Allow the breath to the side of the ribs right here where my fingers are and then relax the breath from here as well' as an example.

Comments

With this release, keep the sense of what is happening at the broadest level possible – periosteum and fascia. Don't be concerned if there is no clear contact with the pectoralis minor. The release here will often be dramatic, with great feelings of openness, a dropped shoulder and floating ribs. These responses are not dependent on a 'direct hit'. In that way it's just like the lateral pterygoid where literal contact may not happen yet the entire region will open in response.

SUBSCAPULARIS

Client

Supine. The arm is abducted to around 45° to allow access to the posterior portion of the axilla. Initially, the arm is placed with the hand resting on the abdomen.

Therapist

Standing at the client's side, at the mid-thoracic level.

Technique

With the forearm supinated so the palm is facing the ceiling, use the tips/pads of the first three fingers to contact the rib cage immediately anterior of the anterior fibers of latissimus dorsi. This is the most posterior aspect of the axilla. Sink medially and contact both the soft tissues and the periosteum of the ribs (Fig. 13.3). Make the contact as broad as possible. Now direct the fingertips in a posterior and medial direction so that they extend into the pocket that lies between the anterior surface of the scapula and the ribs. The pads contact the ribs throughout the release. The tips will be up against the anterior surface of the scapula.

Figure 13.3
Access to the subscapularis via the posterior aspect of the axilla.

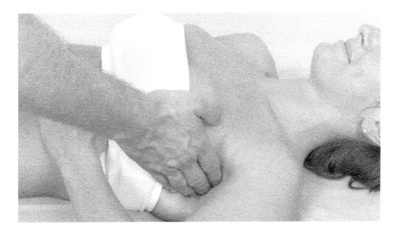

Movement

Have the client slowly introduce external rotation of the shoulder. This should be done mindfully as pain is a likely outcome if the movement is abrupt. At some point before full external rotation is achieved there will be a clear sense of end range being reached. Have the client return the arm to the starting position by controlled internal rotation and repeat the motion into external rotation. Encourage exploration of the motion barrier with two or more movement excursions.

Comments

Occupational demands have led to an increase in carpal tunnel syndrome and other peripheral neuropathies. Some studies on the neurostructural syndrome known as double crush suggest a need to address compression in the whole myofascial complex of the neck, arm and hand rather than only at the periphery. The soft tissue releases for the axillary zone described here are important components of addressing these nerve compressions.

LATISSIMUS DORSI (AT INFERIOR ANGLE OF SCAPULA)

Client

Supine with the arm abducted to 90° and externally rotated so the dorsum of the hand is resting comfortably on the table.

Therapist

Standing at the client's side, at mid-thoracic level.

Technique

Use fingertips or the MP joints of the first two or three fingers to engage the fibers of the latissimus just inferior to the inferior angle of the scapula. Sink through the soft tissue to take the contact through to the ribs (Fig. 13.4). Take up a line of tension in a posterior direction and ask the client to further abduct their arm.

Figure 13.4
Lengthening the latissimus dorsi muscle via contact at its tendinous attachment at the inferior angle of the scapula.

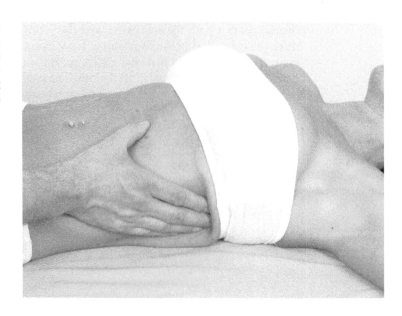

Movement

This can be a similar movement to that for the subscapularis. Having the client explore the motion barrier is rarely painful so fuller abduction will be possible. Explore initiating the movement on the exhale and reducing the effort: 'As you exhale, spread your fingers open and elongate through the bones of your arm to the wall behind your head' as an example.

BRACHIAL FASCIA

Client

Supine, with the arm abducted to 110° and externally rotated so that the dorsum of the hand is resting comfortably on the table.

Therapist

Standing at the client's side, at the mid-thoracic level, and facing superiorly.

Technique

With the palm turned toward the floor, lightly palpate the medial aspect of the humerus between the triceps and biceps (Fig. 13.5). This is done so as to clearly locate the neurovascular bundle and be certain that it is *not* being compressed. Once an unobstructed path to the bone is established, sink through with the fingerpads onto the periosteum. The thumb contacts the lateral arm and a light grasping motion is then developed. Now ask the client to further abduct the arm. Continue the light grasping/squeezing motion.

Figure 13.5
Opening the brachial
fascia.

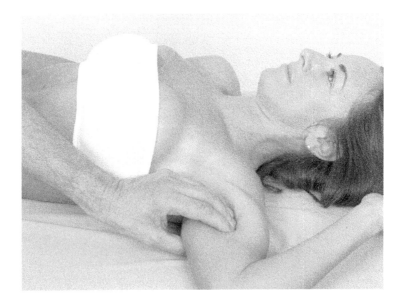

Movement

Abduction of the shoulder is the basic movement. Tension in the fascia will develop close to the end range, often only in the last few degrees. Now ask for rotation of the head to the contralateral side.

Comments

Any nerve sensation, either local or in the hand and fingers, is a sign to stop and reposition. When positioning the client's arm, allow for the level of function and/or pain they have. An arm that cannot be externally rotated will benefit from the support of a pillow or bolster underneath the forearm. This leaves the tissues sufficiently off stretch to allow for entry into the deeper myofasciae.

DEEPER PORTION OF PECTORALIS MAJOR

Client

Supine with the shoulder internally rotated initially, then opening into external rotation.

Therapist

Standing on the ipsilateral side, at the level of the head, facing medial/inferiorly. As the release progresses, turn and face more inferiorly.

Technique

Use the first three fingers of both hands in a stable position to contact the pectoralis major immediately medial to the humeral head (Fig. 13.6). If the fingers hyperextend, use an elbow. Sink directly posterior into the space between the humerus and the rib cage. Engage the first layer of restriction to further posterior motion and wait. When softening occurs, follow this down to the next layer, and so on. Once the deeper layers are accessed, add a line of tension along the course of the space between the ribs and the humerus – lateral/inferior. Take this line to the inferior edge of the pectoralis, which is the anterior boundary of the axilla.

Figure 13.6
Working a deeper layer of release in the pectoralis major.

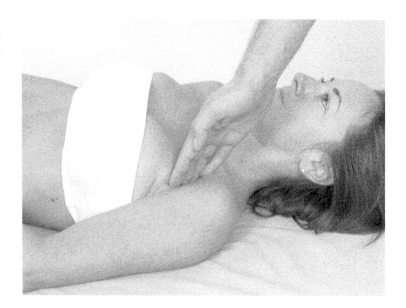

Movement

The first contact is with the client passive. Awareness of the relationship between the exhalation and release in the soft tissue can be verbally encouraged. When the line of tension is developed, the release can be augmented by asking for external rotation and abduction of the shoulder. 'On the exhale, elongate through the arm so the shoulder drops down ... now open the arm away from the body and reach slowly over your head' as an example.

Comments

Use this where an 'upper crossed syndrome' is being addressed. An additional movement that can impact on that syndrome is to have the client retract their scapula during the release. This can be coached with the direction to 'flatten the shoulder into the table' or 'lightly squeeze the shoulder blades together to open the chest'.

The contact is directly over the nerves of the brachial plexus. It is designed, amongst other things, to relieve the tension of the investing fascia of pectoralis minor and the suspensory ligament of the axilla on these nerves. Due to the depth of the intervening tissues which buffer the impact, some nerve sensation is acceptable. However, if nerve sensation is elicited, do not maintain this for longer than 30 seconds. This can lead to unpleasant feelings of neural bruising that can take several days to clear.

Include this release when working with peripheral neuropathies, including carpal tunnel syndrome.

CONOID AND TRAPEZOID LIGAMENTS

Client Supine. The arm is internally rotated with the hand resting on the abdomen.

Therapist Standing at the side of the table at the client's shoulder level.

Technique Rest the pad of the thumb directly onto the coracoid process. Wrap the hand around the shoulder so the contact is spread through the thumb, web, palm and fingers (Fig. 13.7a). Pay attention to not bending the thumb backwards and damaging the joint. Now use the heel of the other hand to apply pressure onto that thumb (Fig. 13.7b). In this way, the upper hand applies movement and

Figure 13.7
Working with the conoid and trapezoid ligaments. **(a)** Initial thumb position. **(b)** Using the other hand to provide the mobilizing force onto the stable thumb.

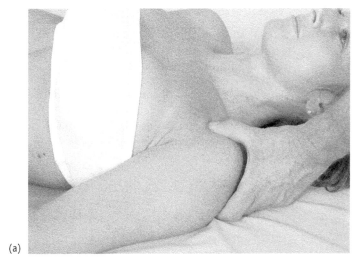

(a)

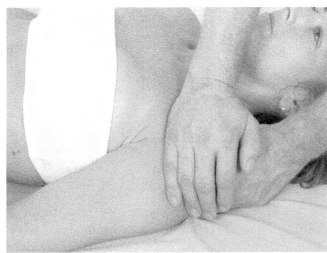

(b)

pressure through the stable thumb onto the coracoid process. Now depress the coracoid posteriorly until resistance to further motion is encountered. Maintain the pressure at this end zone until a palpable softening occurs. If a release is not forthcoming, add a slight pumping motion. Do not allow for a full release of pressure between each pumping action. Rather, oscillate in a zone that is close to the end range so that tension is maintained in the ligaments and fascia throughout the technique.

Movement

This is essentially a passive procedure for the client. Some appropriate comment about the discomfort can be useful. Point out that this type of ligament release is sometimes painful although the pain should be within tolerance. Watch out for stoical, non-verbal responses to pain and adjust the intention accordingly.

Comments

Use this when releasing the short and tight components of an upper crossed syndrome. Consider it as a way to awaken proprioception around the shoulder for any forms of rehabilitation.

FIBROUS RESTRICTIONS AT THE SHOULDER JOINT

Client

Supine. Initially, the shoulder is internally rotated with the palm of the hand resting on the abdomen. External rotation and abduction of the shoulder are introduced during the release.

Therapist

Standing at the head of the table, facing the feet.

Technique

Use a soft fist or an elbow to take up a contact on the medial aspect of the humeral head and the most proximal portion of the humerus (Fig. 13.8). Establish a connection onto the periosteum. Take the line of tension lateral and inferior.

Figure 13.8
Using an elbow to broadly release the shoulder region.

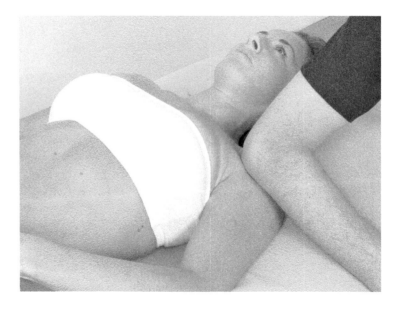

Movement

Have the client introduce external rotation of the shoulder. Make multiple passes while the client continues to actively increase the amount of external rotation. The last few passes can be taken as far as the elbow. Also ask for the head to rotate to the contralateral side.

Comments

With client participation this is a powerful way to get at the fibrous build-up around the shoulder joint. It has a broad effect on the brachial fascia. The distal portion of the release can focus on the biceps brachii and transition across the elbow into that muscle's insertion on the tuberosity of the radius.

All these releases for the shoulder area are important aspects of the treatment of peripheral neuropathies, such as carpal tunnel syndrome. Restrictions in the brachial nerve and its branches can occur at two or more sites that are distant from the symptomatic area. This phenomenon of multiple compressions to the nerve is referred to as double crush syndrome. MFR provides a useful and conservative treatment in this syndrome. Systematic treatment of the soft tissue all the way from the cervical spine to the hand is a good response to the condition rather than attempting to isolate one site as the culprit. The conservative nature of this work is once again stressed. Adopting a systematic approach from the scalenes to the palmar aponeurosis is often useful, sometimes profoundly so. Rarely, if ever, is there a negative outcome. Sometimes no gain is made in the resolution or management of the neuropathy but this is not catastrophic.

THE ELBOW

Client

Supine. The arm is externally rotated at the shoulder and supinated at the elbow. Use a bolster if there is a flexion contracture or any other impediment to the elbow resting in extension.

Therapist

Standing to the side of the table, or seated in a chair, at the client's shoulder level and facing the ipsilateral hand.

Technique

1. Locate the tendon of the biceps brachii where it approaches its insertion into the tuberosity of the radius. Sink into the myotendinous juncture and take up a distal line of tension (Fig. 13.9). Proceed very slowly with attention to

Figure 13.9
Working the area of the elbow via the biceps insertion at the radius.

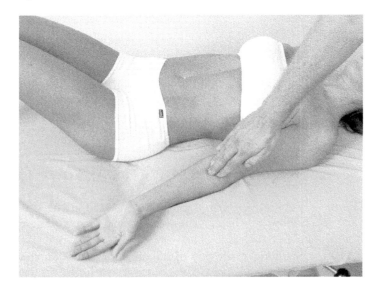

melting the tissues. Adding small twisting motions that increase fascial loading in more than one plane can assist in the opening.

2. Locate the medial epicondyle and contact the shaft of the humerus superior to it (Fig. 13.10). Use the fingertips/pads to sink into the bone and engage the periosteum, without overpressure. Maintain this engagement and slowly work distally onto the epicondyle and then beyond it. The range of movement is slight – less than 5 cm. The client's movement will open the joint.

Figure 13.10
Releasing the elbow via the periosteum of the epicondyle.

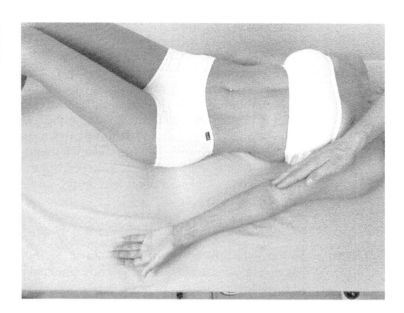

Movement

1. Stabilize the contact and ask the client to slowly pronate the arm while extending the elbow. Now have them twist the arm in the other direction – supination. Alternate between the two movements within a micro range.

2. Have the client extend their fingers and wrist. Coordinate this with their exhale as well as a sense of direction to improve the quality of movement.

Comments

The anatomy of the forearm is detailed and the releases described here are only part of what might be done. Study a good anatomy book and you can start to develop your own approaches. If the basic protocols of engagement are followed a multitude of useful techniques can be developed. It can even be useful to have the anatomy book alongside while you work so that your touch can get quite detailed.

FLEXOR MUSCLES OF THE FOREARM (Fig. 13.11)

Client

Supine. The arm is externally rotated at the shoulder and supinated at the elbow. The hand is off the table and wrist is a fulcrum point at the table's edge.

Therapist

Standing at the side of the table, or seated on chair, at the client's waist level and facing superiorly.

Figure 13.11
The superficial flexor muscles of the left forearm, the palmar aponeurosis and the digital fibrous flexor sheaths (from Baldry PE 2001 Myofascial pain and fibromyalgia syndromes, with permission from Churchill Livingstone).

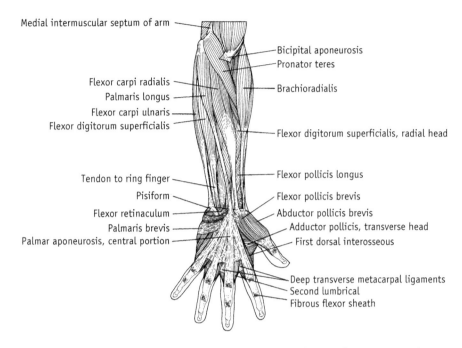

Medial intermuscular septum of arm
Bicipital aponeurosis
Pronator teres
Flexor carpi radialis
Brachioradialis
Palmaris longus
Flexor carpi ulnaris
Flexor digitorum superficialis
Flexor digitorum superficialis, radial head
Tendon to ring finger
Flexor pollicis longus
Pisiform
Flexor pollicis brevis
Flexor retinaculum
Abductor pollicis brevis
Palmaris brevis
Adductor pollicis, transverse head
Palmar aponeurosis, central portion
First dorsal interosseous
Deep transverse metacarpal ligaments
Second lumbrical
Fibrous flexor sheath

Technique

1. Work from distal to proximal. Use an elbow, fist or fingers to sink into the soft tissue on the ulna just proximal to the wrist (Fig. 13.12). Take up a proximal line of tension. Once the tissue is well engaged, have the client

Figure 13.12
Releasing the forearm flexors via the ulna.

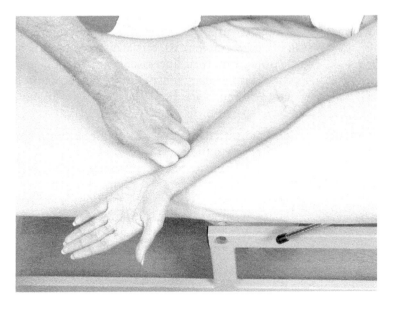

further supinate their arm against the moderate resistance of your pressure. Make a number of contacts along the edge of the ulna, moving towards the elbow. The more proximal portion is done with the fingers to allow access to the bone behind the large flexor digitorum profundus muscle.

2. Work from proximal to distal. Start on the medial epicondyle of the humerus. Use the elbows or fingerpads to work into the broad muscles of the forearm: pronator teres, flexors carpi radialis and ulnaris, and flexor digitorum superficialis (Fig. 13.13). Take up a line of tension in a distal direction and ask for supination as well as wrist and finger extension.

Figure 13.13
Releasing the broad muscles of the forearm: pronator teres, flexors carpi radialis and ulnaris, and flexor digitorum superficialis.

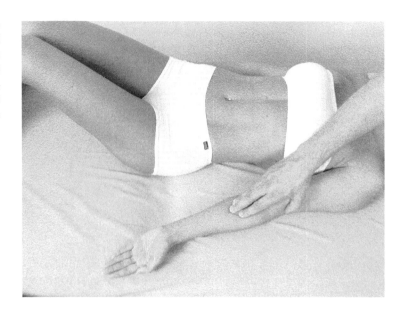

Movement   Give the client a specific direction of movement: 'Turn the thumb towards the floor' as an example. An effective micro movement is to have the client 'play the piano' with their fingers and explore subtle motion in each finger. This, of course, brings many muscles of the forearm into play; perhaps its real significance is in the awareness of the discrete joyful motion available in the fingers.

Comments   Equipped with the knowledge of double crush syndrome, all sites of potential compression should be assessed via palpation and treated according to the finding. The median nerve and ulnar artery pass beneath the origin of flexor digitorum superficialis. Give attention to this zone when working with peripheral neuropathies. With these conditions, some relief should be experienced in the first session although resolution or reduction of symptoms may require multiple treatments over several months. Altering work habits and addressing ergonomics are essential to obtain long-lasting outcomes.

PALMAR ASPECT OF THE HANDS (Fig. 13.14)

Client   Supine. The arm is externally rotated at the shoulder and supinated at the elbow.

Therapist   Standing to the side of the table at the level of the elbow and facing toward the hand.

Figure 13.14
Superficial dissection of
muscles of the palm of the
right hand (from Baldry PE
2001 Myofascial pain and
fibromyalgia syndromes,
with permission from
Churchill Livingstone).

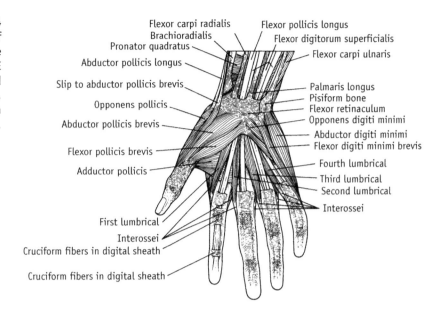

Flexor carpi radialis
Brachioradialis
Pronator quadratus
Abductor pollicis longus
Slip to abductor pollicis brevis
Opponens pollicis
Abductor pollicis brevis
Flexor pollicis brevis
Adductor pollicis
First lumbrical
Interossei
Cruciform fibers in digital sheath
Cruciform fibers in digital sheath

Flexor pollicis longus
Flexor digitorum superficialis
Flexor carpi ulnaris
Palmaris longus
Pisiform bone
Flexor retinaculum
Opponens digiti minimi
Abductor digiti minimi
Flexor digiti minimi brevis
Fourth lumbrical
Third lumbrical
Second lumbrical
Interossei

Technique

1. Use the fingerpads or the pad of a well-supported thumb to take up a contact on the flexor retinaculum (transverse carpal ligament) at its medial attachment (Fig. 13.15). Put in a line of tension in a lateral direction (toward the thenar eminence). Hold the tension in the tissue while the client adducts their thumb, thus taking it away from the point of contact. Carry the line of tension in a lateral/distal direction (just medial to the mound of the thenar eminence and into the webbing).

Figure 13.15
Release of the
flexor retinaculum, flexor
pollicis brevis, abductor
pollicis brevis and
opponens pollicis.

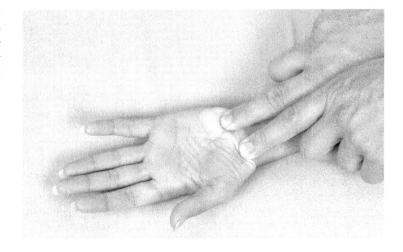

2. Turn the client's hand over into pronation. Clasp both your hands over the dorsum of their hand so that your fingers can reach around to meet on the palmar surface of their hand (Fig. 13.16a). Apply your weight through your thenar eminences so you cause the client's hand to be pushed into your

Figure 13.16
Palmar fascia release.
(a) Two-handed approach.
(b) Finger position.

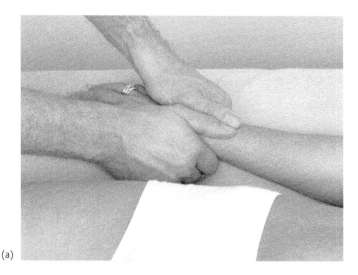

(a)

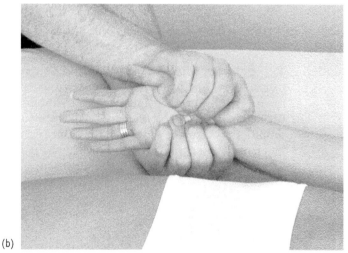

(b)

fingers. Apply a twisting and wringing motion between your hands that puts movement into their carpal bones. Move the contact further into the center of the palm and apply the same twisting and wringing actions while simultaneously spreading your fingertips away from each other (Fig. 13.16b).

Movement

1. This is essentially a technique to bring release to the muscles of the thenar eminence: flexor pollicis brevis, abductor pollicis brevis and opponens pollicis. Any action of the thumb that brings awareness to the area will be helpful.
2. The twisting motions will assist with mobilizing the carpal bones as well as releasing tensions in the interossei and lumbricals. This aspect of the release is generally highly pleasurable.

Comments

The retinaculum, the transverse carpal ligament, is the origin of both the opponens pollicis and opponens digiti minimi. All the oppositional actions between the thumb and fifth metacarpal put strain here. This is pressuring the carpal tunnel. Overuse of the grasping actions, particularly as used in the kneading strokes of massage, generates ongoing compression of the median nerve as it passes through the tunnel. This can lead to subclinical conditions that in time give way to a full breakdown in hand function. I recommend minimizing the grasping action of massage as an essential step in the prevention of initial or further problems.

Given the contemporary epidemic of carpal tunnel syndrome, all this talk of peripheral neuropathies and so on is important but it would be unfortunate to leave it only at the level of rehabilitation. Consider all the emotional meanings of holding hands – love, trust and care. Work in the hand is some of the most delightful that there is. Done slowly, and with an appreciation of the PNS, it leads to deeply pleasurable and system-wide release. Work around the hand is an excellent starting point for rebalancing the ANS. Use it as a prelude to cranial work, for instance, to get a rapid shift in ANS function.

TRICEPS

Client

Supine with the ipsilateral shoulder flexed to 110° and the elbow flexed to 90°. The palm is resting on the table; if this is not comfortable, add a pillow to raise the hand from the table and reduce the amount of shoulder flexion.

Therapist

Standing at the head of the table.

Technique

1. Treat from distal to proximal. Palpate on either side of the triceps tendon until it becomes possible to reach under the muscle and make a contact between it and the bone. The fingertips of each hand are pointed at each other under the muscle, in effect slightly lifting it up off the humerus (Fig. 13.17). A proximal line of tension is developed and carried as close to the scapula as possible. Subsequent passes will allow the fingers to move more under the muscle.

Figure 13.17
Triceps release:
two-handed approach.

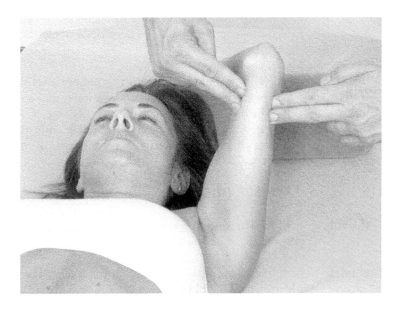

2. Palpate and isolate the long head of the triceps tendon at the scapula. Sink against the periosteum and simultaneously capture the tendon (Fig. 13.18). Tether firmly without overpressure.

Figure 13.18
Treating the long head of the triceps at the scapula.

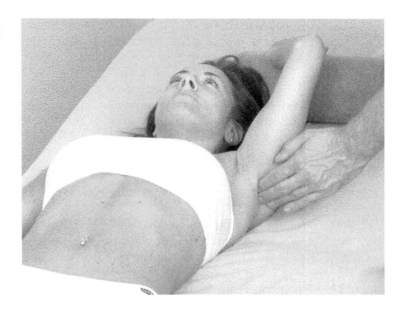

Movement

1. Coach the client to lengthen through the humerus in counterpoint to your proximal line of tension. As the hand is resting on the table or pillow, there is a closed chain situation that gives a definite sensation of reaching into something solid. This makes the proprioceptive awakening much greater than simply reaching can do. Further coaching can encourage a sense of moving the humerus without automatically engaging the scapula. This is best accomplished with a micro movement with verbal encouragement from the therapist to leave the scapula resting on the table.
2. The movement is essentially the same as for the first release. A fuller, more macro movement can also be developed while the tendon is tethered against the bone.

Comments

Triceps, for some reason, don't get much attention although they're often hypertonic, stringy and inelastic. When treating any shoulder joint restriction, always include these two releases. This is true even when the primary restriction is clearly on the anterior aspect of the joint. Working in this manner, on both sides of a joint, is a good approach with all MFR.

EXTENSOR MUSCLES OF THE FOREARM

Client

Supine. The shoulder is internally rotated, the elbow pronated and flexed to around 15°. The palm is resting flat on the table.

Therapist

Standing to the side of the table at the level of the client's shoulder and facing the ipsilateral hand.

Technique

1. Begin on the humerus, just proximal to the lateral epicondyle. Use the elbow, fingertips or soft fist to engage the periosteum (Fig. 13.19). Carry this contact inferior to the common extensor tendon and then down to the extensor retinaculum of the wrist.

Figure 13.19
Treating from the common extensor tendon to the extensor retinaculum of the wrist.

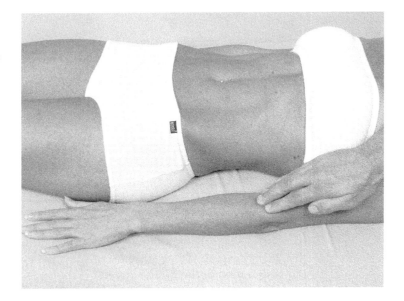

2. Use the fingerpads or knuckles to work the periosteum of the ulna (Fig. 13.20).

Figure 13.20
Using the fingerpads to work the periosteum of the ulna.

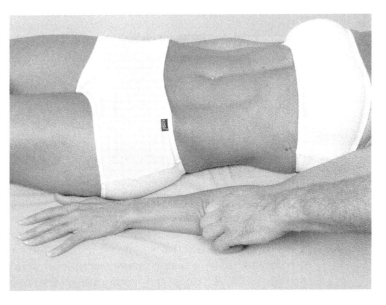

3. Contact the head of the ulna with the fingerpads of one hand and the dorsal tubercle of radius with the pads of the other (Fig. 13.21). Engage through to the periosteum and put a line of tension in a lateral and distal direction. This is carried for just a few centimeters with a firm intent to 'spread' the bones apart.

Figure 13.21
Spreading the radius from the ulna.

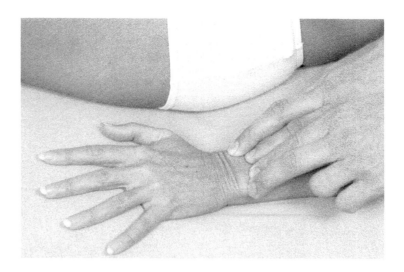

Movement

1. Coach the client to slowly flex and extend the elbow within an easy range of 5–10°. Use this motion to generate more multiplanar shearing forces in the myofascia. Resist the motion but do not prevent it.
2. While engaging the periosteum of the ulna, ask for alternating ulnar and radius deviation of the hand.

Comments

Working in the arm, especially around the elbow and wrist, produces strong release in the respiration. Watch for a number of deep, spontaneous therapeutic breaths.

The initial intention should be at the surface, with a lot of multiplanar fascial shearing. After mobility and responsiveness are established, take the work deeper. Slow, patient work here will open up the posterior interosseous membrane. You will feel the radius and ulna float free in the soft tissue when this happens.

DORSUM OF HAND

Client

As above.

Therapist

As above.

Technique

This is an extension of the release made in technique 3, above. Start proximal to the carpal bones. Use the fingerpads to take up a line of tension across the extensor retinaculum of the wrist. Carry this onto the carpal bones, metacarpals and phalanges. Give sufficient compressive force to squash the hand into the treatment table in such a manner as to produce a pleasant feeling of pressure (Fig. 13.22). Done several times, this will lead to a feeling of the carpal bones being mobilized.

Movement

Easy, unpressured ulnar and radial deviation can be helpful.

Comments

Just as with the releases in the palmar surface of the hand, watch for changes in overall ANS activity. Changes in respiratory function will be observed. The

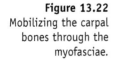
Figure 13.22
Mobilizing the carpal
bones through the
myofasciae.

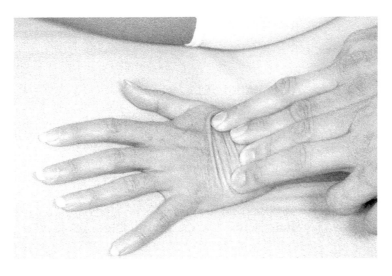

only complaint that many therapists, particularly the very serious ones, have
when they do this work on each other in my classes is that it feels too good to
be considered therapeutic. Hmmm…

Inflammatory disorders such as arthritis are often considered contraindications for soft tissue therapies. This is reasonable given that the outcome of
therapy is highly variable and a significant number of people experience an
exacerbation of their symptoms post treatment. Introducing this work into the
arthritic hand is worth considering. Explore the possibility of using MFR in
these situations by introducing small amounts – less than 10 minutes – of very
low force MFR and then get feedback about the response over the next
24 hours. This amounts to a low-risk experiment which may show that MFR
provides real relief. With a small amount of input only, the downside would be
a slight flare-up that creates a minimum of distress.

Introducing small amounts of MFR is like using the titration tubes in the
chemistry lab. Drop by measured drop is delivered until the exact amount
required for success arrives. Following this model means patience and follow-
up. I've personally found that many arthritic clients have responded to MFR
titrated in this way, as have people with chronic fatigue and fibromyalgia.

PEDIATRIC SUPPLEMENT FOR THE UPPER EXTREMITIES

It is necessary to develop a stable pelvis and trunk before doing detailed work
on the arms. Release of the proximal arm structures should precede work in
the distal aspect. Without adequate release and control of the shoulder joint,
there will be minimal gain from working the hand and elbow. Clear restrictions
in the shoulder girdle, cervical and upper thoracic areas prior to attempting
release on the arms. While work in the distal extremities is helpful for provoking useful change in the ANS, it is my clinical observation that this is not the
case with CP infants and children. Without trunk stability, MFR in the distal
upper extremity is not that productive.

At the shoulder, address the two most consistently restricted areas – the
hypertonic and stiff subscapularis and pectoralis minor. For the most part,

modifying these releases for a pediatric setting is a matter of scale. Often it is just a single finger doing the release.

SUBSCAPULARIS

Client

Generally supine but sidelying position can also be used (shown here).

Therapist

Position is dependent on the treatment surface.

Technique

Use one hand to abduct the scapula so the axillary border moves laterally, away from the ribs. Use the first two fingers of the other hand at the posterior section of the axilla to sink against the upper ribs (Fig. 13.23). Next, take these fingertips posteriorly so that the anterior surface of the scapula is contacted. To avoid activation of the SNS, the contact is spread as broadly as possible.

Figure 13.23
Releasing the subscapularis in sidelying position.

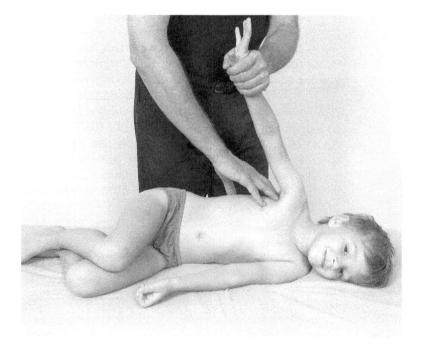

Movement

The child's initial involuntary action may be contraction. Don't be put off by this but maintain a moderate, firm contact and wait for a release. Once that is established, ask for a movement. If active movement is not possible, use passive motion.

Comments

This release will influence much more than simply the subscapularis. Think of the intrafascial mechanoreceptors and their relationship to the CNS and ANS. Possible components of the release will include the ribs, breathing, the pleura and the cervical myofascia.

PECTORALIS MINOR

Client

Supine. The arm is bolstered if necessary to put the tissues off stretch.

Therapist

As for above.

Technique

Use one or possibly two fingers to engage the ribs at the anterior section of the axilla. Next, while maintaining a clear contact with the ribs, move the fingers under the pectoralis major up against the lateral aspect of pectoralis minor (Fig. 13.24). Keep the contact broad and maintain it until an obvious cycle of release is completed. This may take up to 2 minutes.

Figure 13.24
MFR to the
pectoralis minor.

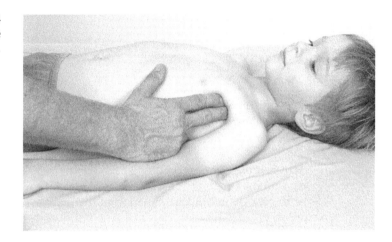

Movement

Once again, the initial response may be contraction. Once this passes, it becomes possible to explore active, or passive, movement. However, as with adults, it's highly likely that movement will increase the sensation to a painful level. This is to be avoided. Sensations of softening and lowered tone are more important than mobilizing the tissue with movement.

Comments

This release will also influence the surrounding myofasciae.

ELBOW FLEXORS

Client

Supine, with the arm fully supported so the flexor muscles of the elbow are not on stretch. This is very important.

Therapist

Depends on the treatment surface.

Technique

Use the first two fingers of one hand to engage the distal section of the medial shaft of the humerus. Sink between the bone and the biceps to engage the medial intermuscular septum of the arm (Fig. 13.25). Work proximal to distal,

Figure 13.25
Release to the
intermuscular septa
of the elbow region.

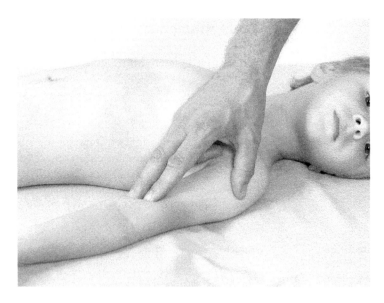

across the epicondyle and into the lower arm. Carry the line of tension along the lateral aspect of pronator teres and sink into the intermuscular septum of the lower arm. This can be approximated by sinking under the biceps tendon.

Movement   Active elbow extension should be encouraged although this is often not possible with the CP child. Passive motion is useful. However, the initial goal should be to provide maximal stimulation of the mechanoreceptors via sustained firm pressure.

Comments   As stated above, it's important to position the arm so that the MFR can be done without provoking a stretch. Without an initial response in the fascia, passive stretching will be of no value.

TRICEPS

Client   Variable. Supine works well when the arm is fixed in adduction, internal rotation and elbow flexion. Sidelying works when fixed trunk flexion makes supine position difficult.

Therapist   Depends on the treatment surface. Shown here on a table. Note the attention to a clear line of support through the fingers and wrist. This allows for an obvious sense of directed intention.

Technique   Use the pad of one or possibly two fingers to palpate and isolate the long head of the triceps tendon at the scapula (Fig. 13.26). Sink against the tendon and then on into the periosteum. Engage firmly without overpressure.

Movement   Active 'reaching' motions if possible; passive movement is useful.

Figure 13.26
MFR to the triceps.

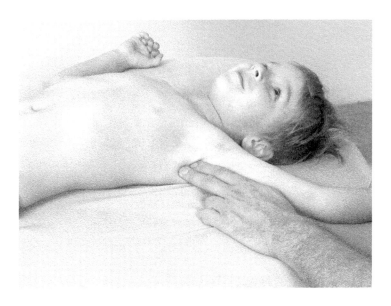

Comments The most common condition I find in CP children is arm in adduction, internal rotation, elbow and wrist flexion. It may seem counterintuitive to release the triceps. However, if direct technique MFR is seen as a means to provide sensory stimulation via the mechanoreceptors, and not a simple lengthening procedure, treating the triceps makes more sense. Control at the shoulder and elbow joints requires balanced action on both sides of the joints. Therapists are encouraged to use this triceps release and observe the outcome. It will improve the controls rather than destabilizing them. For the rationale behind this strategy, see the section on neuromotor control in Chapter 2.

INDEX

Printed and bound by CPI Group (UK) Ltd, Croydon, CR0 4YY

03/10/2024

01040366-0016